Managing Depression in Clinical Practice



For other titles published in this series, go to
www.springer.com

# Managing Depression in Clinical Practice

Edward S Friedman and Ian M Anderson

With contributions from

Danilo Arnone
Timothey Denko

Springer

Edward S Friedman
Associate Professor of Psychiatry
University of Pittsburgh School of Medicine
Director, Mood Disorders Treatment and Research Program
Western Psychiatric Institute and Clinic
Pittsburgh, USA

Ian M Anderson
Professor of Psychiatry
Neuroscience and Psychiatry Unit
Mental Health and Neurodegeneration Research Group, School of Medicine
University of Manchester
Manchester
UK

*With contributions from*
Danilo Arnone, DM
Clinical Training Fellow
University of Manchester
Manchester, UK

Timothey Denko, MD
Western Psychiatric Institute and Clinic
Pittsburgh, PA, USA

ISBN 978-1-84996-464-7 e-ISBN 978-1-84996-465-4
DOI 10.1007/978-1-84996-465-4

A catalogue record for this book is available from the British Library

Library of Congress Control Number: 2010935583



Springer Science+Business Media
springer.com

# Contents

# Author biographies

Edward S Friedman, MD, received his Doctor of Medicine degree from the University of Pittsburgh School of Medicine in Pittsburgh, Pennsylvania, USA. Upon graduation, he joined the faculty of the University of Pittsburgh School of Medicine Department of Psychiatry and the Western Psychiatric Institute and Clinic (WPIC) of the University of Pittsburgh Medical Center. Currently, he is the Director of the Mood Disorders Treatment and Research Program at WPIC. His research has focused on cognitive behavioral psychotherapy, pharmacotherapy, and combination treatments for major depression and bipolar illness. He has published numerous articles and book chapters on these subjects. Recently, he was the National Cognitive Therapy Director for the landmark STAR*D study. Dr Friedman is also Director of the Cognitive Therapy Residency Training Program and the Ambulatory Mood and Anxiety Disorders Residency Training Program at WPIC. Dr Friedman has participated in many mood disorders research projects, and, for example, he is currently the Pittsburgh site Primary Investigator for the National Institute of Mental Health Depression Treatment Network and the National Institute of Mental Health Bipolar Treatment Network – multicenter collaborations that have been responsible for the highly-regarded STEP-BD and STAR*D studies.

Professor Ian M Anderson is a Professor of Psychiatry at the University of Manchester and an Honorary Consultant Psychiatrist at Manchester Mental Health and Social Care Trust. He studied medicine at Cambridge University and University College Hospital Medical School, going on to training posts in general medicine and neurosurgery before training in psychiatry in Oxford. He is Director of the Specialist Service for Affective Disorders in Manchester, which he founded in 2001 as a multidisciplinary tertiary service for treatment-resistant depression and bipolar disorder. His current research interests concern the role of serotonin in the etiology and treatment of affective disorders and the use of functional brain imaging to investigate emotional processing and neurotransmitter function in depression. He is first author of the British Association for Psychopharmacology (BAP) guidelines for treating depressive disorders with antidepressants, and a co-author of the BAP guidelines for treating anxiety disorders. He was Chair of the Clinical Guideline Development Group to update the National Institute for Health and Clinical Excellence treatment guideline for depression.

# Preface

Is there a need for yet another book about depression? This is the question we asked ourselves in the planning stages of this book. Given that you are now reading this preface, we obviously thought there was—but why? Developments in the field are currently evolutionary rather than revolutionary but new treatments do become available, old and new treatments are reevaluated, and patient choice and the structure of treatment delivery are increasingly emphasized. This means that there is a need for updated accessible summaries for those who need to keep abreast of current thinking and apply their knowledge in practice. As our backgrounds are from both sides of the Atlantic, we have tried to keep both perspectives in mind. We have had to be necessarily brief and emphasize areas that we believe are important. Inevitably we have had to skate over complexities, but we have tried not to oversimplify and to provide key references for further reading. Although primarily aimed at nonspecialists and students, we hope that for more experienced practitioners this book also provides a useful overview of the subject.

# Chapter 1

## Classification, causes, and epidemiology

Edward S Friedman

### Different types of depression

The depressive disorders comprise a heterogeneous group of illnesses that are characterized by differing degrees of sad mood and associated cognitive, neurovegetative, and psychomotor alterations. Depression is currently the fourth most disabling medical condition in the world and it is predicted to be second only to ischemic heart disease with regard to disability by 2020 [1,2].

#### Depressive disorders

There is a broad spectrum of depressive disorders characterized by the presence of sad mood and varying degrees of other depressive symptoms [3]. According to the American Diagnostic and Statistical Manual of Mental Disorders, 4th edition (DSM-IV) [4], disturbance of mood is the predominant feature of mood disorders. They are further divided into the bipolar disorders (characterized by the presence of a manic or hypomanic episode – which may also include depressive episodes, hence the older term manic depression) and the depressive disorders. The latter are subdivided into major depressive disorder (MDD) and dysthymic disorder (DD), as well as a "not otherwise specified" category for subsyndromal cases that do not fulfill the criteria for MDD or DD. MDD is characterized by one or more major depressive episodes (MDEs) – a period during which an individual experiences five or more depressive symptoms to a moderate degree for 2 weeks or longer with a diminution of their previous level of functioning (see Figure 1.1). In addition, these symptoms cannot be attributed to another psychiatric or medical disorder, the direct physiologic effect of a substance, or bereavement. In circumstances where an individual presents with sad mood and clinically significant impairment, the term "depressive disorder not otherwise specified" is used.

The *International Classification of Mental and Behavioral Disorders*, 10th revision (ICD-10) [5] characterizes recurrent depressive disorder as repeated

E. Friedman and I.M. Anderson, *Managing Depression in Clinical Practice*
DOI 10.1007/978-1-84996-465-4_1, © Springer-Verlag London Limited 2010

## Characterization of a major depressive disorder

| ICD-10 classification | | DSM-IV classification | |
|---|---|---|---|
| Criteria symptoms: at least 2 weeks of lowered mood*, anhedonia*, reduced energy*, reduced concentration, sleep disturbances, reduced appetite, reduced self-confidence, feelings of guilt and worthlessness, psychomotor retardation or agitation, loss of libido | | Criteria symptoms: at least 2 weeks of low or depressed mood*, anhedonia*, significant changes in appetite, disturbed sleeping patterns, psychomotor retardation or agitation, reduced energy levels, feelings of guilt and worthlessness, reduced concentration/decision making, ideas or acts of self harm or suicide | |
| * Most typical (ICD-10) or core (DSM-IV) symptoms | | | |
| Depressive episode | | Major depressive disorder, single episode | |
| Mild: 4 symptoms including at least 2 of the most typical symptoms and some difficulty in continuing with usual activities | F32.0 | Mild severity: few if any symptoms beyond 5 (including at least one core symptom); mild level of disability or the capacity to function normally but with substantial and unusual effort | 296.21 |
| Moderate: 5 or 6 symptoms including at least 2 of the most typical symptoms; usually considerable difficulty in continuing with usual activities | F32.1 | Moderate severity: severity and disability intermediate between mild and severe | 296.22 |
| Severe: at least 7 symptoms, some severe, including all 3 of the most typical symptoms; very unlikely that that the sufferer can continue with usual activities | F32.2 | Severe: several symptoms beyond 5 (including at least one core symptom); with clear-cut, observable disability | 296.23 |
| Severe with psychotic features: as F32.2, with psychotic symptoms (e.g., delusions, hallucinations and stupor) | F32.3 | Severe with psychotic features: as 296.23, with psychotic symptoms (e.g., delusions or hallucinations) | 296.24 |
| Other<br>Includes atypical depression | F32.8 | Unspecified | 296.20 |
| Unspecified | F32.9 | In partial remission: some symptoms of MDE are present but full criteria no longer met; or there are no longer any significant symptoms but period of remission is less than 2 months in duration | 296.25 |
| | | In full remission: ≥2 months without any symptoms | 296.26 |

| ICD-10 classification | | DSM-IV classification | |
|---|---|---|---|
| Recurrent depressive disorder | | Major depressive disorder, recurrent | |
| Mild: at least one previous episode, current episode as F32.0 | F33.0 | Mild: at least one previous episode, current episode as 296.21 | 296.31 |
| Moderate: at least one previous episode, current episode as F32.1 | F33.1 | Moderate: at least one previous episode, current episode as 296.22 | 296.32 |
| Severe: at least one previous episode, current episode as F32.2 | F33.2 | Severe: at least one previous episode, current episode as 296.23 | 296.33 |
| Severe with psychotic features: at least one previous episode, current episode as F32.3 | F33.3 | Severe with psychotic features: At least one previous episode, current episode as 296.24 | 296.34 |
| Other | F33.8 | Unspecified | 296.30 |
| Unspecified | F33.9 | In partial remission: at least one previous episode, current episode as 296.25 | 296.35 |
| Currently in remission: at least two previous episodes, but has had no symptoms for several months | F33.4 | In full remission: at least one previous episode, current episode as 296.26 | 296.36 |

Figure 1.1 Characterization of a major depressive disorder. MDE, major depressive episode. Adapted from [4] and [5].

episodes of depression without any history of independent episodes of mood elation and hyperactivity. They subdivide the depressive episode category according to severity as being mild (at least two of the most typical symptoms of depression and two other symptoms), moderate (at least two of three most typical symptoms of depression and three or four other symptoms), or severe (all three most typical symptoms of depression and at least four other symptoms) (Figure 1.1). ICD-10 also accepts duration of symptoms of less than 2 weeks if the symptoms are unusually severe or of rapid onset.

There are several subtypes of depression that are described in the DSM-IV as specifiers to denote that they are subcategories of MDEs:

- *Dysthymia* describes a less severe, chronic, and persistent disorder. The DSM-IV diagnosis of dysthymia requires depressed mood to be present for most of the day, nearly every day, for a period of more than 2 years. The symptoms of dysthymic disorder differ from those of MDD by slower onset, longer duration and persistence, and lower severity. The mildest forms of depression are sometimes termed "subsyndromal depression."
- *Chronic* describes an MDE of more than 2 years in duration.

- *With melancholic features* describes a condition of extremely severe anhedonia – the almost complete loss of interest in and lack of reactivity to usually pleasurable activities. In addition, there must be three or more of the following features:
  - a distinct quality of depressed mood that differs from the kind of feeling following a loss
  - depression that is worse in the morning
  - early morning awakening
  - marked psychomotor agitation or retardation
  - significant appetite and/or weight loss
  - inappropriate or excessive guilt.
- *Catatonic features* describes an MDE with at least two of the following:
  - catalepsy or stupor
  - excessive and purposeless motor activity
  - postural rigidity or mutism
  - posturing, stereotyped movements, prominent mannerisms, or grimacing
  - echolalia or echopraxia.
- *Atypical features* denotes the presence of mood reactivity; i.e., the ability for the depressed individual's mood to brighten in response to actual or potential positive events, along with two or more of the following:
  - hyperphagia
  - hypersomnia
  - leaden paralysis
  - a long-standing pattern of interpersonal rejection sensitivity that results in significant social or occupational impairment (a trait with an early onset that persists throughout life).
- *Psychotic features*: the presence or absence of such features is specified according to whether they are consistent with depressive themes, termed "mood-congruent features," as opposed to mood-incongruent features, which are less common – persecutory delusions, thought insertion/withdrawal delusions, thought broadcasting, or control delusions. Furthermore, the *onset* of an MDE can be described by the presence or absence of preceding *dysthymia* or *postpartum* status if the episode begins within 4 weeks of delivery.
- *Seasonal features* describes a course of depressive illness characterized by specific onset and remission of symptoms associated with characteristic times of the year. Most commonly, depressive symptoms manifest in fall/autumn and/or winter and spontaneously remit in spring or summer. To qualify for this diagnosis, in the last 2 years there must be two MDEs

demonstrating a temporal relationship and the individual cannot have more nonseasonally than seasonally related MDEs.

Several outcomes have been described to characterize an individual's treatment trajectory (see Figure 8.1). The most serious consequence of depression is the increased risk of suicide; for example, Bostwick and Pankratz [6] examined patients with affective disorders and estimated the lifetime prevalence of suicide in those hospitalized with suicidal ideation as 8.6% and for those hospitalized without suicidal ideation as 4.0%. The lifetime suicide prevalence for mixed inpatient/outpatient populations was 2.2%, and for the nonaffectively ill population less than 0.5%. These data demonstrate that there is an increased risk of suicide with increasing intensity of suicidal ideation and suggest that suicide risk increases with depressive illness severity.

## Causes of depression

Dualistic theories separating mind and brain are being replaced with more integrated models that consider the biological, psychological, and social influences that produce depression. Kandel's understanding of mind–brain interactions provides a model for understanding the nature and possible causes of depression [7], particularly:

- All mental processes derive from the brain.
- Genes and their protein products determine neuronal connections and functioning.
- Life experiences influence gene expression and psychosocial factors feed back to the brain.
- Altered gene expression that produces changes in neuronal connections contributes to maintaining abnormalities of behavior.
- Psychotherapy produces long-term behavior change by altering gene expression.

Therefore, both genetic and environmental factors are implicated in the etiology and treatment of depression. Recent advances in the study of the genetic basis of depression have produced interesting findings, such as a functional polymorphism of the serotonin transporter gene, which can be used to predict selective serotonin reuptake inhibitor (SSRI) response in the context of life stress [8]. Thus, depression can be understood to be the consequence of life stress interacting with heritable genetic and personality vulnerabilities that produce physiological and psychological dysfunction.

The prolonged exposure to stress produces characteristic alterations in brain neurotransmitter function often described as a "chemical imbalance."

This refers to alterations in the major chemical messenger systems responsible for neuronal transmission: serotonin (5HT), norepinephrine/noradrenaline (NE), and dopamine (DA). Depression has been associated with reductions in neurotransmission in these systems and currently available antidepressant medications are thought to work by reversing these deficits [9]. The alterations in these neuronal systems produce the characteristic psychological and somatic symptoms characteristic of depression (see Chapter 3).

Other theories of the etiology of depression derive from the perspectives of their discipline; e.g., the interpersonal theory examines interpersonal stress and role transition as causes of depression. The cognitive model posits that dysfunctional thoughts foster depression and reinforce behaviors that promote the depressive state. The dynamic model focuses upon unconscious psychological conflict with the goal of the individual achieving insight or needed support. One very interesting model has been proposed by Brown and colleagues (Figure 1.2), who describe mechanisms responsible for the onset, provocation, and perpetuation of depression [10]. A "severe life event" can provoke the onset of an MDE. Proximal risk factors mediate the onset of the depressive episode, and distal risk factors both mediate the proximal risk factors and foster the perpetuation of a chronic illness course.

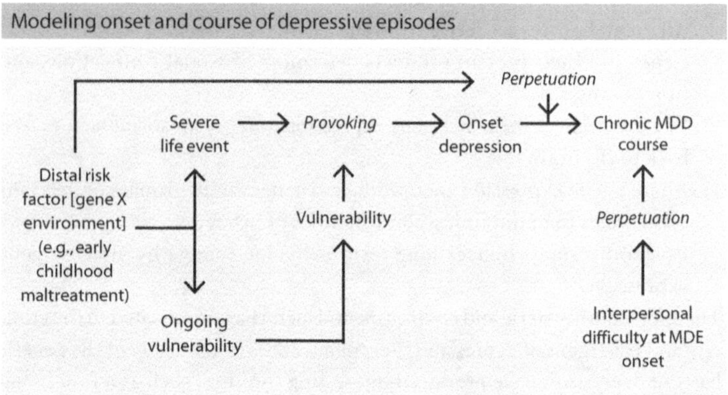


Figure 1.2 Modeling onset and course of depressive episodes. This model proposes mechanisms that are responsible for the onset, provocation, and perpetuation of depression. A "severe life event" can provoke the onset of a major depressive episode (MDE). Proximal risk factors (e.g., a poor quality interpersonal relationship) mediate the onset of the depressive episode. Distal risk factors (e.g., early childhood maltreatment) both mediate the proximal risk factors (life events and ongoing vulnerabilities) and foster the perpetuation of a chronic illness course. Adapted from [10].

In addition, there are many medical diseases that commonly manifest with symptoms of depression (Figure 1.3), and many drugs can also produce depressive symptoms as adverse effects (Figure 1.4). Several other psychiatric diseases can also present with symptoms of depression, including schizophrenia, anxiety disorders, eating disorders, and substance abuse.

| Diseases commonly associated with depressive symptoms | |
|---|---|
| Brain trauma/brain tumor | Lyme disease |
| Cancer (especially pancreatic) | Multiple sclerosis |
| Cardiovascular disease | Normal pressure hydrocephalus |
| Dementia | Parkinson's disease |
| Diabetes | Pellegra |
| Epilepsy | Porphyria |
| HIV/AIDS | Rheumatoid arthritis |
| Huntington's disease | Stroke |
| Hyperthyroidism | Syphilis |
| Hypothyroidism | Systematic lupus erythematosus |
| Hyperparathyroidism | Wilson's disease |
| Hypoparathyroidism | |

Figure 1.3 Diseases commonly associated with depressive symptoms

| Drugs that may cause depression | |
|---|---|
| Anticancer agents | Hormones |
| Interferon-α | Estrogen |
| Vincristine sulfate | Progesterone |
| Vinblastine sulfate | |
| | Opioids |
| Antihypertensive agents | Codeine |
| Clonidine hydrochloride | Morphine |
| Guanethidine sulfate | |
| Methyldopa | Alcohol |
| Propranolol hydrochloride | |
| Reserpine | Anticholinergics |
| | Benztropine |
| Antiparkinsonian agents | |
| Amantadine hydrochloride | Barbiturates |
| Bromocriptine | Phenobarbital |
| Levodopa | Secobarbital |
| Levodopa and carbidopa | |
| | Benzodiazepines |
| Antituberculosis agents | |
| Cycloserine | |
| Corticosteroids | |
| Cortisone acetate | |

Figure 1.4 Drugs that may cause depression

## Epidemiology and natural history

MDD is a highly prevalent disorder. The most recent US estimates of the prevalence were 16.2% for lifetime and 6.6% for the 12 months before the survey. The age of onset varies with birth cohorts (Figure 1.5), with a fairly low risk until the teenage years, after which it rises in a linear fashion, and more steeply in more recent age cohorts. Prevalence seems to be lower outside the US and varies between countries, but global rates are still high, with one meta-analysis of 23 studies from countries across Europe, Asia, North and South America, and Australasia finding pooled rates of 6.7% lifetime prevalence and 4.1% 12-month prevalence [11]. Depressive disorders are the fourth most important cause of disability worldwide, and are expected to become the second most important cause by 2020 [1,2]. Sociodemographic correlates of increased risk of MDD in the USA include age, female gender, nonwhite race/ethnicity, employment status, not being married, having less education, lower income, and urbanicity. Nearly all MDD respondents reported at least some role impairment and three-quarters of respondents with lifetime MDD reported at least one comorbid medical disorder [12]. A recent representative clinical sample has revealed that MDD is often chronic, severe, and with substantial clinical comorbidity; for example, two-thirds of individuals in the large Sequenced Treatment Alternatives to Relieve Depression (STAR*D) effectiveness study reported at least one concurrent general medical condition [13]. MDD is usually an episodic disorder with an episode occurring on average every 5 years; however, 20–33% of individuals suffer a chronic and unremitting course [14]. Those individuals who do not achieve a complete remission of symptoms are more likely to experience a relapse [13,15]. Longer depressive episodes appear to be more difficult to treat and individuals with low levels of depressive symptoms are about three times more common than individuals with MDD level symptoms [16].

Approximately 20–33% of patients who experience an MDE have a course defined by early onset and chronic dysthymic course [17]. The National Comorbidity Survey of the US population found a 12-month prevalence of 2.5% for dysthymia with a lifetime prevalence of 6.4%, and about 3% for chronic depression [18]. Individuals with chronic major depression experience an earlier age of onset, increased axis II comorbidity, likelihood of experiencing an early trauma history, and genetic familial loading for depressive illness, less effective coping strategies, more chronic stress, less social support, marked impairment in psychosocial function and work performance, and increased healthcare utilization [19–21].

MDD with melancholic features is distributed equally among men and women, and is more likely in older individuals and those experiencing psychotic features (DSM-IV). Atypical features are twice as common in women as in men, and individuals with these features have an earlier age of onset and a more persistent, less episodic, and more chronic course (DSM-IV).

Postpartum depression is the most common complication of childbearing and occurs in 13% of women after delivery [22]. The prevalence of winter-type seasonal depression varies with increased rates with higher latitude and younger age. Women make up 60–80% of those with this disorder (DSM-IV).

Cumulative lifetime prevalence of CIDI/DSM-IV major depressive disorder by birth cohort

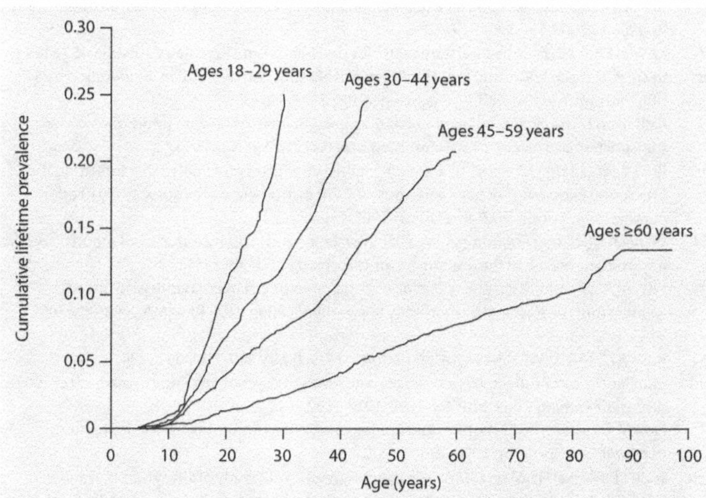


Figure 1.5 Cumulative lifetime prevalence of CIDI/DSM-IV major depressive disorder by birth cohort. CIDI, Composite International Diagnostic Interview. Adapted with permission from [12].

## References


1 Murray CJ, Lopez AD. Alternative projections of mortality and disability by cause 1990–2020: global burden of disease study. Lancet 1997; 349:1498–1504.

2 Lopez AD, Mathers CD. Measuring the global burden of disease and epidemiological transitions: 2002–2030. Ann Tropical Med Parasitol 2006; 100:481–499.

3 Remick RA, Sadovnick AD, Lam RW, et al. Major depression, minor depression, and double-depression: are they distinct clinical entities? Am J Med Genet 1996; 67:347–353.

4 American Psychiatric Association. The Diagnostic and Statistical Manual of Mental Disorders, 4th ed. Washington DC: APA, 1994.

5 World Health Organization. International Classification of Mental and Behavioral Disorders, 10th revision (ICD-10). Geneva: WHO, 1992.

6 Bostwick JM, Pankratz VS. Affective disorder and suicide risk: a reexamination. Am J Psychiatry 2000; 157:1924–1932.

7 Kandel ER. A new intellectual framework for psychiatry. Am J Psychiatry 1998; 55:457–469.

8 Caspi A, Sudgen K, Moffitt TE, et al. Influence of life stress on depression: moderation by a polymorphism in the 5-HTT gene. Science 2003; 301:386–389.

9 Richelson E. The clinical relevance of antidepressant interaction with neurotransmitter transporters and receptors. Psychopharmacol Bull 2002; 36:133–150.

10 Brown WG, Craig TKJ, Harris TO. Parental maltreatment and proximal risk factors using the Childhood Experience of Care and Abuse (CECA) instrument: a life course study of adult chronic depression – 5. J Affect Disord 2008; 110:222–233.

11 Waraich P, Goldner EM, Somers JM, et al. Prevalence and incidence studies of mood disorders: a systematic review of the literature. Can J Psychiatry 2004; 49:124–138.

12 Kessler RC, Berglund P, Demler O, et al. The epidemiology of major depressive disorder: Results from the National Comorbidity Survey Replication (NCS-R). JAMA 2003; 289:3095–3105.

13 Rush AJ. STAR*D: What have we learned? Am J Psychiatry 2007; 164:201–204.

14 Mueller TI, Leon AC. Recovery, chronicity, and levels of psychopathology in major depressive disorder. Psychiatr Clin North Am 1996; 19:85–102.

15 Fava M, Davidson KG. Definition and epidemiology of treatment-resistant depression. Psychiatr Clin North Am 1996; 19:179–200.

16 Judd LL, Akiskal HS, Maser JD, et al. A prospective 12-year study of subsyndromal and syndromal depressive symptoms in unipolar major depressive disorders. Arch Gen Psychiatry 1998; 55:694–700.

17 AHCPR Depression Guideline Panel. Clinical Practice Guideline. Number 5. Depression in Primary Care, vol 1. Detection and Diagnosis. Rockville, MD: US Department of Health and Human Services, Public Health Service, Agency for Health Care Policy and Research, 1993.

18 Kessler RC, McGonagle KA, Zhao S, et al. Lifetime and 12-month prevalence of DSM-III-R psychiatric disorders in the United States. Results from the National Comorbidity Survey. Arch Gen Psychiatry 1994; 51:8–19.

19 Keller MB, McCullough JP, Klein DN, et al. A comparison of nefazodone, the cognitive behavioral-analysis system of psychotherapy, and their combination for the treatment of chronic depression. N Engl J Med 2000; 342:1462–1470.

20 Nemeroff CB, Heim CM, Thase ME, et al. Differential responses to psychotherapy versus pharmacotherapy in the treatment of patients with chronic forms of depression. Proc Natl Acad Sci USA 2003; 100:14293–14296.

21 Schatzberg AF, Rush AJ, Arnow BA, et al. Chronic depression: medication (nefazodone) or psychotherapy (CBASP) is effective when the other is not. Arch Gen Psychiatry 2005; 62:513–520.

22 O'Hara MW, Swain AM. Rates and risk of postpartum depression: a meta analysis. Int Rev Psychiatry 1996; 8:37–54.

# Chapter 2

## Depression in different types of patients

Timothey Denko and Edward S Friedman

### Depression in children

Depression has been estimated to have a prevalence in children of 2.5% and in adolescents of 4–8% [1]. The presentation of symptoms of depression in young people is, to a large extent, similar to that of adults, especially with respect to the presence of neurovegetative symptoms of depression. Decline in psychosocial performance (primarily in school) and reduced interest in previously enjoyed activities may be more easily detected signs that a younger individual is experiencing symptoms of depression. In addition, irritability may be more common in depressed children and adolescents than in depressed adults.

In 2003, the UK Medicine and Healthcare products Regulatory Agency (MHRA) concluded that all SSRIs, with the exception of fluoxetine, were contraindicated in the treatment of depression in young people, due to an increase in suicidal ideation, as well as dubious efficacy. In 2004, the US Food and Drug Administration (FDA) issued a "black box warning" concerning an increased risk of suicidal ideation and behavior in people under the age of 18 treated with second-generation antidepressants.

The primary analysis of randomized controlled trials (RCTs) of SSRIs that led to the FDA "black box warning" revealed an increase over baseline of roughly 2% (placebo 2% versus 4%) in suicidal ideation or behavior in people under the age of 18 given an SSRI. No children completed suicide in the RCTs included in this analysis. The difference in suicidal ideation leads to a number needed to harm (NNH) of 50. A subsequent meta-analysis of 27 RCTs of SSRIs in children and adolescents with depression, obsessive–compulsive disorder, and other anxiety disorders [2] again found no completed suicides and a smaller increase in suicidal ideation/self harm attempts with SSRIs, corresponding to an NNH of 143. The validity of using "suicidality" (meaning suicidal behaviour, ideation, or attempts) as a surrogate for suicide, as in these studies, has been criticized [3], given the relatively high incidence of suicidality in comparison to

E. Friedman and I.M. Anderson, *Managing Depression in Clinical Practice* 
DOI 10.1007/978-1-84996-465-4_2, 

completed suicide. Studies of the efficacy of SSRIs in children and adolescents suggest a number needed to treat (NNT) of 5 for fluoxetine and 9 for SSRIs overall [4]. The Texas Medication Algorithm Project (TMAP) [5] considers fluoxetine, citalopram, and sertraline to be first-line medications for treatment of depression in children and adolescents, and the relatively small increase in suicidal ideation to be less significant than the benefit from treating them with SSRIs. Fluoxetine is the most highly recommended, and is still the only FDA-approved SSRI for the treatment of depression in those aged under 18. Paroxetine should be avoided in pre-adolescents.

Second-generation antidepressants such as bupropion, venlafaxine, duloxetine, and mirtazapine have little evidence to support their use in children and adolescents, and should be considered second- or third-line choices for pharmacologic treatment: the younger the child, the less the therapeutic benefit gained from second-generation antidepressants.

Alternatively, evidence-based psychotherapies such as cognitive–behavioral therapy (CBT) are also recommended, either singly or together with medication, in the treatment of depression in younger people. The combination of fluoxetine and CBT showed the most robust response in the Treatment of Adolescents with Depression Study (TADS) when compared with CBT alone or fluoxetine alone in moderately to severely depressed adolescents [6]. Fluoxetine outperformed CBT alone in this study. However, other studies [7–9] have found the combination of CBT and an SSRI to have no greater efficacy than the SSRI alone.

## Depression in elderly people

The prevalence of MDDs (i.e., meeting full DSM-IV criteria) is thought to decrease with increasing age [10]. Unfortunately, rates for completed suicide increase with advancing age, to the point that people over the age of 86 have the highest suicide rate of any age group [11]. Medical burden, loss of loved ones, decreased independence, and financial hardship are thought to contribute to the likelihood of a depressive episode in elderly people.

There are difficulties in diagnosing depression in elderly people because they tend to report somatic complaints much more readily than sad mood. Other cardinal symptoms of depression, such as sleep disturbance and/or alterations in appetite or energy, can also be nonspecific changes that are common in normal aging. Depression is often comorbid with cardiovascular disease in elderly adults, and it has been suggested that circulatory problems can actually cause depressive symptoms, possibly by affecting the flow of blood to the brain. This type of depression has been termed "vascular depression," although this disorder is not yet recognized by the standard guidelines. *Clinically significant depression* is a category meant to capture older adults with less than full DSM-IV depressive episodes, but still meaningful depression. This diagnosis is thought to be much more common than MDD. Symptoms that can aid in identifying the depressed older adult include decreased interest (anhedonia) and social withdrawal in individuals who were previously engaged and interested in activities. Treatment in this age group is discussed in Chapter 4.

## Depression in women

Women have close to twice the lifetime prevalence of depressive disorders of men [10]. Nearly all of this increased susceptibility to depression occurs during the childbearing years, from menarche to menopause. A number of variables, both psychosocial and biological, may contribute to these disparate rates of depression. As increased rates of depression in women follow ovarian function closely, estrogen has been extensively studied as a mediator of depression in women, and is, therefore, a potential agent for the treatment of depression. To date, studies of estrogen in the treatment of depression in perimenopausal and postmenopausal women have not yielded consistent findings of benefit, and ovarian hormones are not included in standard treatment recommendations for this group [12].

Depression during pregnancy can be difficult to detect, because many of the neurovegetative signs of depression are common in pregnancy. The rate of depression in pregnant women is thought to be similar to that of non-pregnant women. *Postpartum depression* follows one in eight deliveries, and can be differentiated from the benign "baby blues" by duration and severity of symptoms, and the negative impact on maternal psychosocial function. Conversely, the "baby blues" should be limited to 10 days after delivery, and psychosocial functioning should be reasonably preserved. The treatment of postpartum depression mirrors the treatment of standard depression.

Outside the reproductive-cycle–associated increase in prevalence of depression in women, few other compelling differences have been identified when comparing depression in women and men. In the STAR*D study, clinical characteristics of 2541 outpatients with major depression were compared by gender. Two-thirds of the sample were women. Women had greater symptom severity but men had more MDEs. Women were found to have greater rates of an anxiety disorder, bulimia, and somatoform disorders, as well as more suicide attempts, whereas men showed more alcohol and substance use disorders. Irritability was equally common in men and women [13].

## Depression in patients with comorbid medical conditions

Depressive disorders occur more frequently in people with chronic medical conditions, and are associated with poorer long-term outcomes. Disorders of the central nervous system (CNS), such as Parkinson's disease, dementia, cerebrovascular disease (post-stroke depression [PSD], vascular dementia), and multiple sclerosis all have strong associations with depressive disorders. Chronic medical illnesses not directly affecting the CNS, such as human immunodeficiency virus (HIV), cancer, coronary artery disease, and autoimmune disorders have also been associated with higher rates of depressive disorders (see Figure 1.3). Identifying a mediator and a direction of association for these findings has been difficult.

PSD is estimated to occur in approximately a third of patients within 9 months of having a cerebrovascular accident (CVA). It can be difficult to diagnose and can mimic symptoms of depression; for example, individuals with aphasia are unable to complete a clinical interview; individuals with anosognosia may be unaware of their deficits; or individuals with physical limitations that impair the ability to engage in hedonic activities may seem to be anergic. PSD is related to poor functional outcomes, as well as poor cognitive outcomes, and its successful treatment is thought to lead to significant improvement in both cognition and function.

Depression has been linked to cardiovascular disease, as both a risk factor for developing heart disease and a predictor of increased mortality in patients with heart disease. Mediators of such an association may include inflammatory cytokines, increases in platelet thrombus formation, or alterations in sympathetic and parasympathetic tone to the cardiac conduction system.

Depression is estimated to occur in 24% of patients diagnosed with cancer. Of course, this is a highly heterogeneous group representing many types of malignancies. Pancreatic, head and neck, and breast cancer appear to have the highest rates of associated depression. Factors that can affect the emergence of depressive disorders can include the severity of the illness, disfigurement, and effects of treatment – surgical, radiation, or chemotherapeutic. Conversely, as depression is thought to lower immune system function, people with depression may be at higher risk for cancer. Successful treatment of depression in these populations can improve quality of life as well as medical outcome.

## References


1 Ford T, Goodman R, Meltzer H. The British Child and Adolescent Mental Health Survey. J Am Acad Child Adolesc Psychiatry 2009; In press.
2 Klein DF. The flawed basis for FDA post-marketing safety decisions: the example of anti-depressants and children. Neuropsychopharmacology 2006; 31:689–699.
3 Bridge JA, Iyengar S, Salary CB, et al. Clinical response and risk for reported suicidal ideation and suicide attempts in pediatric antidepressant treatment: a meta-analysis of randomized controlled trials. JAMA 2007; 297:1683–1696.
4 Usala T, Clavenna A, Zuddas A, et al. Randomized controlled trials of selective serotonin reuptake inhibitors in treating depression in children and adolescents: a systematic review and meta-analysis. Eur Neuropsychopharmacol 2008; 18:62–73.
5 Crismon ML, Trivedi MH, Pigott TA, et al.; for the Texas Consensus Conference Panel. The Texas Medication Algorithm Project: report of the Texas consensus conference panel on medication treatment of major depressive disorder. J Clin Psychiatry 1999; 60:142–156.
6 TADS Team. The Treatment for Adolescents With Depression Study (TADS): Long-term effectiveness and safety outcomes. Arch Gen Psychiatry 2007; 64:1132–1435.
7 Clarke G, Debar L, Lynch F, et al. A randomized effectiveness trial of brief cognitive-behavioral therapy for depressed adolescents receiving antidepressant medication. J Am Acad Child Adolesc Psychiatry 2005; 44:888–898.
8 Melvin GA, Tonge BJ, King NJ, et al. A comparison of cognitive-behavioral therapy, sertraline, and their combination for adolescent depression. J Am Acad Child Adolesc Psychiatry 2006; 45:1151–1161.
9 Goodyer I, Dubicka B, Wilkinson P, et al. Selective serotonin reuptake inhibitors (SSRIs) and routine specialist care with and without cognitive behaviour therapy in adolescents with major depression: randomized controlled trial. BMJ 2007; 335:142.
10 Kessler RC, Berglund P, Demler O, et al. The epidemiology of major depressive disorder: results from the National Comorbidity Survey Replication (NCS-R). JAMA 2003; 289:3095–3105.
11 Karch D, Lubell K, Friday J, et al. Surveillance for violent deaths – national violent death reporting system, 16 states 2005. MMWR Surveill Summ 2008; 57:1–45.
12 Aloysi A, Van Dyke K, Sano M. Women's cognitive and affective health and neuropsychiatry. Mt Sinai J Med 2006; 73:967–975.
13 Marcus, SM, Kerber KB. Sex differences in depression symptoms in treatment-seeking adults: confirmatory analyses from the Sequenced Treatment Alternatives to relieve Depression study. Compr Psychiatry 2008; 49:238–246.

# Chapter 3

# Diagnosis

Edward S Friedman

## Signs and symptoms of depression

Depression is characterized by symptoms that generally fall into two categories: psychological, and somatic or physical. The former are characterized by a persistent sense of sadness, termed "dysphoria," and a persistent state of lack of usual enjoyment or pleasure in previously pleasurable activities, termed "anhedonia." Depressed individuals with dysphoria describe themselves as being helpless and hopeless, discouraged, "blue," "fed up," or "down in the dumps" and "useless." They are often easily tearful, irritable, or frustrated because they tend to have negatively biased perceptions about themselves and others to whom they relate, and a pessimistic view of their future, often manifesting as inappropriate guilt. The most serious symptom of depression with respect to mortality and morbidity is suicidal behavior [1]. The most benign type of suicidal thinking – that "life is not worth living" – is consonant with beliefs by individuals that their lives are hopeless, they are helpless and worthless, and have no chance for future betterment. Suicidal thinking around plans to harm oneself (or others) indicates a higher level of potential risk, which is greatest when the individual is contemplating acting on the plans or has demonstrated behavior in furtherance of the suicidal thinking. Proximal risk factors for suicide include agitation, current suicidal intent or plan, severe depression and/or anhedonia, instability (e.g., alcohol abuse or decline in health), recent loss, and availability of a lethal agent. Distal risk factors include current suicidal intent with plan, personal or family history of suicide, aggressive or impulsive behavioral pattern (including possible bipolar disorder, especially if associated with psychosis), poor response to treatment for depression, poor treatment alliance, a history of abuse or trauma, and/or substance or alcohol abuse [2]. The most common risk factors for suicide are summarized in Figure 3.1 [3].

E. Friedman and I.M. Anderson, *Managing Depression in Clinical Practice*
DOI 10.1007/978-1-84996-465-4_3, 

| Risk factors for suicide:"sad persons" scale | |
|---|---|
| S | Sex: more than three males for every female kill themselves |
| A | Age: older > younger, especially white males |
| D | Depression: a depressive episode precedes suicide in up to 70% of cases |
| P | Previous attempt(s): most people who die from suicide do so on their first or second attempt. Patients who make multiple (≥4) attempts have increased risk of future attempts rather than suicide completion |
| E | Ethanol use: recent onset of ethanol or other sedative–hypnotic drug use increases the risk and may be a form of self-medication |
| R | Rational thinking loss: profound cognitive slowing, psychotic depression, pre-existing brain damage, particularly frontal lobes |
| S | Social support deficit: may be result of the illness that can cause social withdrawal |
| O | Organized plan: always need to inquire about presence of a plan when treating a depressed patient |
| N | No partner: again, may be a result rather than a cause of the depressive disorder, but nevertheless absence of a partner or significant other is a risk factor |
| S | Sickness: intercurrent medical illnesses |

Figure 3.1 Risk factors for suicide: "sad persons" scale. Reprinted with permission from Preskorn [3].

Somatic symptoms of depression include alterations from normal sleep, termed "insomnia" when reduced (mild if <30 min, moderate if <120 min, and severe if >120 min to fall asleep) and, when increased, termed "hypersomnia" (mild if >30 min, moderate if >30 but <120 min, and severe if >120 min). Insomnia is often described by when it occurs in the sleep cycle: difficulty in falling asleep, sleep continuity disturbance or midnight awakening, and early morning awakening. Unusual increases or decreases in appetite are common, as well as corresponding fluctuations in weight. Psychomotor changes may manifest as psychomotor activity: agitation, anxiety, and/or hyperactivity. Less frequently, individuals may present with psychomotor retardation: decreased activity, slowed thought processes, and a reduction in content and process (mutism) – termed "catatonia" in its extreme presentation. Some individuals report lack of energy and persistent fatigue, often accompanied by lack of motivation and inability to initiate tasks.

The ICD-10 system considers sad mood, anhedonia, and reduced energy leading to fatigue to be the three typical symptoms of depression. The other common symptoms of depression include reduced concentration or attention, reduced self-esteem and self-confidence, ideas of guilt and worthlessness, a pessimistic view of the future, thoughts of self-harm or suicide, disturbed sleep, and decreased appetite. The classification for a depressive episode in the DSM-IV and ICD-10 systems are summarized in Figure 1.1.

## Differential diagnosis

Depressive episodes must be differentiated from other general medical conditions (DSM-IV category mood disorders due to a general medical condition), substance-induced mood disorders (DSM-IV substance-induced mood disorder), and other psychiatric disorders.

Other medical conditions that may present with symptoms characteristic of depression are listed in Figure 1.3, and include cerebrovascular, endocrine, metabolic, neurological, and infectious disorders. In addition, more than half of the depressed individuals in the ecologically valid STAR*D study reported co-occurring general medical conditions [4]. If there is such a general medical disorder and the MDD is not judged to be the direct physiological consequence of this condition, DSM-IV suggests coding the MDD as the psychiatric disorder and the general medical condition as a medical disorder, suggesting no etiological connection between the two conditions.

Individuals may present with symptoms characteristic of depression caused by ingestion of a drug of abuse, medication, or toxin – DSM-IV substance-induced mood disorders. Figure 1.4 lists common medications that can produce depressive symptoms. Individuals who present with depressive symptoms while using drugs of abuse, such as cocaine, methamphetamine, and opioids, require detoxification to determine if there is a co-occurring depressive episode before a depressive diagnosis can be made. The very common condition of co-occurring mood and substance abuse disorders is termed "dual diagnosis." For DSM, if the depressed mood occurs only in the context of withdrawal from a substance, it is considered substance-induced mood disorder with depressive features.

Other psychiatric illnesses may also present with signs and symptoms associated with depression. In its acute presentation, a depressive disorder with mood-congruent psychotic features, hallucinations, and/or thought disorder may be difficult to distinguish from schizophrenia or schizoaffective disorder. Other information, such as illness history and course, the individual's premorbid history, and family history, may aid in making a differential diagnosis. Due to cognitive impairment, dementia may also be difficult to distinguish from depression. Often, depression in elderly people can be masked by dementia (i.e., the pseudodementia of depression) and the prominent cognitive impairment resolves with remission of the depressive episodes. On the other hand, dementia must be ruled out in elderly people presenting with depression through medical and laboratory evaluation, an examination of the premorbid history, the commonality of onset of depressive and cognitive symptoms, the course of illness, and the response to antidepressants. Depressive episodes can also be confused with normal grief reactions (termed "bereavement" in DSM-IV) after the death of a loved one. Usually, grief reactions are associated with symptoms of insomnia, poor appetite, and weight loss, and are not associated with decreased self-esteem or suicidal ideation. The duration of normal grieving is culturally determined, but the DSM-IV suggests that, if such symptoms of depression persist for more than 2 months after the loss, the diagnosis of MDD should be considered.

## The patient examination and interview

A proficiently performed psychiatric interview will provide the patient and clinician with a specific and accurate diagnosis, while ideally establishing a caring relationship based on mutual respect and collaboration. The interview should start with an empathic statement by the psychiatrist of the goals of the examination and how that will aid the patient. Inquiring after patients' reasons for the examination in their own words and determining a chief complaint in an empathic and relaxed manner may help put patients at ease and will foster cooperation, which enhances the accuracy of the clinical data obtained.

A history of the present episode should include a complete description of duration, intensity, and extent of the depressive symptoms. To aid in this process, the use of clinical self-assessment instruments can be extremely helpful in gathering this information, as well as for the purposes of monitoring the progress of symptomatic improvement. Figure 3.2 presents one such instrument – the Quick Inventory of Depressive Symptomatology – Self Rated, 16 Items (QIDS-$SR_{16}$) [5] and other rating scales are briefly presented in Figure 4.2. The QIDS-$SR_{16}$ was used in the ecologically valid, large-scale STAR*D study [6] as a component of measurement-based care – the use of depressive measures to determine medication dosage increases and measures of side effects to determine medication dosage reductions (see the STAR*D website at www.edc.gsph.pitt.edu/stard to download the QIDS-$SR_{16}$ and the FISER [Frequency, Intensity and Side Effect Rating] scale). Utilizing such tools, equally good depression outcomes were achieved by psychiatrists and family practitioners. The QIDS-$SR_{16}$ quantifies the somatic and psychological symptoms of depression, including the presence or extent of suicidal ideation and/or planning and intent. In addition, in reviewing the circumstances around the onset of the depressive episode, it is important to inquire about recent life stresses experienced by the patient to help us better understand the psychological and social forces at play in their lives and how these may have affected the onset of the current depressive episode.

## STAR*D QIDS-$SR_{16}$

Choose the response to each item that best describes you for the past 7 days

1. Falling asleep (during the past 7 days ....)
   0 I never take longer than 30 minutes to fall asleep.
   1 I take at least 30 minutes to fall asleep, less than half the time.
   2 I take at least 30 minutes to fall asleep, more than half the time.
   3 I take more than 60 minutes to fall asleep, more than half the time.

2. Sleep during the night (during the past 7 days ...)
   0 I do not wake up at night.
   1 I have a restless, light sleep with a few brief awakenings each night.
   2 I wake up at least once a night, but I go back to sleep easily.
   3 I awaken more than once a night and stay awake for 20 minutes or more, more than half the time.

3. Waking up too early (during the past 7 days ...)
   0 Most of the time, I awaken no more than 30 minutes before I need to get up.
   1 More than half the time, I awaken more than 30 minutes before I need to get up.
   2 I almost always awaken at least 1 hour or so before I need to, but I go back to sleep eventually.
   3 I awaken at least 1 hour before I need to, and can't go back to sleep.

4. Sleeping too much (during the past 7 days ...)
   0 I sleep no longer than 7–8 hours/night, without napping during the day.
   1 I sleep no longer than 10 hours in a 24-hour period, including naps.
   2 I sleep no longer than 12 hours in a 24-hour period, including naps.
   3 I sleep longer than 12 hours in a 24-hour period, including naps.

5. Feeling sad (during the past 7 days ...)
   0 I do not feel sad.
   1 I feel sad less than half the time.
   2 I feel sad more than half the time.
   3 I feel sad nearly all the time.

*Please complete either 6 or 7 (not both)*

6. Decreased appetite (during the past 7 days ...)
   0 There is no change in my usual appetite.
   1 I eat somewhat less often or lesser amounts of food than usual.
   2 I eat much less than usual and only with personal effort.
   3 I rarely eat within a 24-hour period, and only with extreme personal effort or when others persuade me to eat.

*OR*

7. Increased appetite (during the past 7 days ...)
   0 There is no change from my usual appetite.
   1 I feel a need to eat more frequently than usual.
   2 I regularly eat more often and/or greater amounts of food than usual.
   3 I feel driven to overeat both at mealtime and between meals.

*Please complete either 8 or 9 (not both)*

8. Decreased weight (within the last 2 weeks)
   0 I have not had a change in my weight.
   1 I feel as if I have had a slight weight loss.
   2 I have lost 2 pounds or more.
   3 I have lost 5 pounds or more.

Figure 3.2 STAR*D QIDS-$SR_{16}$

## STAR*D QIDS-SR$_{16}$

*OR*

9. Increased weight (within the last 2 weeks)
   0 I have not had a change in my weight.
   1 I feel as if I have had a slight weight gain.
   2 I have gained 2 pounds or more.
   3 I have gained 5 pounds or more.

10. Concentration in decision-making (during the past 7 days ...)
   0 There is no change in my usual capacity to concentrate or make decisions.
   1 I occasionally feel indecisive or find that my attention wanders.
   2 Most of the time, I struggle to focus my attention or to make decisions.
   3 I cannot concentrate well enough to read or cannot make even minor decisions.

11. View of myself (during the past 7 days ...)
   0 I see myself as equally worthwhile and deserving as other people..
   1 I am more self-blaming than usual.
   2 I largely believe that I cause problems for others.
   3 I think almost constantly about major and minor defects in myself.

12. Thoughts of death or suicide (during the past 7 days ...)
   0 I do not think of suicide or death.
   1 I feel that life is empty or wonder if it's worth living.
   2 I think of suicide or death several times a week for several minutes.
   3 I think of suicide or death several times a day in some detail, or I have made specific plans for suicide or have actually tried to take my life.

13. General interest (during the past 7 days ...)
   0 There is no change from usual in how interested I am in other people or activities.
   1 I notice that I am less interested in people or activities.
   2 I find I have interest in only one or two of my formerly pursued activities.
   3 I have virtually no interest in formerly pursued activities.

14. Energy level (during the past 7 days ...)
   0 There is no change in my usual level of energy.
   1 I get tired more easily than usual.
   2 I have to make a big effort to start or finish my usual daily activities (e.g., shopping, homework, cooking, or going to work).
   3 I really cannot carry out most of my usual daily activities because I just don't have the energy.

15. Feeling slowed down (during the past 7 days ...)
   0 I think, speak, and move at my usual rate of speed.
   1 I find that my thinking is slowed down or my voice sounds dull or flat.
   2 It takes me several seconds to respond to most questions and I'm sure my thinking is slowed.
   3 I am often unable to respond to questions without extreme effort.

16. Feeling restless (during the past 7 days...)
   0 I do not feel restless.
   1 I'm often fidgety, wringing my hands, or need to shift how I am sitting.
   2 I have impulses to move about and am quite restless.
   3 At times, I am unable to stay seated and need to pace around.

Figure 3.2 STAR*D QIDS-SR$_{16}$ continued

**STAR*D QIDS-SR$_{16}$**

To score the QIDS-SR$_{16}$

Enter the highest score on any one of the four sleep items (1–4 above):
Enter the highest score on item 5:
Enter the highest score on any one appetite/weight item (6–9):
Enter the highest score on item 10:
Enter the highest score on item 11:
Enter the highest score on item 12:
Enter the highest score on item 13:
Enter the highest score on item 14:
Enter the highest score on either of the two psychomotor items (15 and 16):
Total score (range: 0–27):

QIDS-SR$_{16}$ scoring
6–10 = mild depression
11–15 = moderate depression
16–20 = severe depression
21 or more = very severe depression

Figure 3.2 STAR*D QIDS-SR$_{16}$ continued

The examination should then include a detailed history of past psychiatric illness episodes. Each episode should be assessed for precipitating events, symptomatic intensity and duration, degree of lethality, suicidality, homocidality, or other self-harm behaviors, and the presence of other co-occurring illnesses or conditions. A history of substance and/or alcohol use is also essential.

A review of the patient's personal, developmental, and social history should be undertaken and information should be obtained regarding: childhood developmental delays, early trauma or abuse, and early socialization experiences with friends and in school; family circumstances (i.e., custody or guardianship arrangements); financial and vocational issues; home environment issues; religious and spiritual orientation; and sexual history.

A complete and comprehensive medical history should include active medical problems, current medication(s) (including over-the-counter medications and medications for nonpsychiatric illnesses), past medical history, family medical history, and a medical review of systems.

The mental status (state) examination is a core component of the psychiatric examination. The clinician should note and comment upon the patient's general appearance, general condition, level of motoric activity, and extent of compliance, cooperation, and collaboration in the interview.

Objective signs such as tics, tremors, eye contact, and interactive style should be described. The patterns associated with, and the extent and intensity of dysphoria and anhedonia, and the patient's range of affect, should be noted, and the rate, pattern, and content of speech and thought and the presence of abnormal perceptions described. An assessment of cognitive function is necessary and if cognitive dysfunction is exposed on cursory examination (e.g., being alert and oriented to person, place, time) the use of a standardized measure, such as the Mini-Mental State Examination (MMSE) [7], can be very helpful. If indicated, a referral for formal cognitive testing may be made. Finally, an assessment of the patient's insight into the illness and the quality of judgment should be noted.

## Laboratory tests for co-occurring illnesses

Currently, there are no laboratory tests that can be clinically used to diagnose depression. Laboratory testing is done primarily to rule out other co-occurring medical disorders that may present as depression. In addition, urine and serum laboratory tests are used to screen for substances of abuse or rule out some form of toxicity, which may also mimic the symptoms of depression. Laboratory tests are routinely obtained for hospital inpatient admissions and patients newly diagnosed with a depressive disorder. Figure 1.3 lists common co-occurring medical illnesses with symptoms similar to depression, and Figure 1.4 lists common medications that may cause symptoms similar to depression.

Commonly used laboratory examinations and associated co-occurring medical illnesses are:

- *Complete (full) blood count (CBC) with differential*: anemias, blood dyscrasias, inflammatory disorders, infection.
- *Serum chemistries*: electrolytes, glucose (diabetes), calcium (hyperparathyroidism, arrhythmia), magnesium (neuromuscular and renal disease), liver function tests (hepatic disease), sodium (adrenal function), creatinine, and blood urea nitrogen (renal function).
- *Thyroid function tests*: if thyroid-stimulating hormone (TSH) is abnormal, obtain triiodothyronine ($T_3$), thyroxine ($T_4$), and free hormone concentration (hyperthyroidism or hypothyroidism).
- *Rapid plasma regain (RPR) or Venereal Disease Research Laboratory (VDRL)*: syphilis.
- *Urinanalysis*: screen for renal disorders or metabolic or systemic disease.
- *Urine toxicity screen*: drug or substance of abuse toxicity.
- *Chest X-ray* (patients over 35 years of age): arrhythmia, respiratory dysfunction.
- *Blood toxicity screen or levels of other medications taken* (if indicated): toxicity.

## References


1 Rihmer Z. Suicide risk in mood disorders. Curr Opin Psychiatry 2007; 20:17–22.

2 Hawton K, Harriss L. Deliberate self-harm in young people: characteristics and subsequent mortality in a 20-year cohort of patients presenting to hospital. J Clin Psychiatry 2007; 68:1574–1583.

3 Preskorn SH. Outpatient Management of Depression: A Guide for the Practitioner, 2nd edition. Caddo, OK: Professional Communications Inc, 1999.

4 Yates WR, Mitchell J, Rush AJ. Clinical features of depressed outpatients with and without co-occurring general medical conditions in STAR*D. Gen Hosp Psych 2004; 26:421–429.

5 Rush AJ, Trivedi MH, Ibrahim HM, et al. The 16-item Quick Inventory of Depressive Symptomatology (QIDS), clinician rated (QIDS-C), and self-report (QIDS-SR): a psychometric evaluation in patients with chronic major depression. Biol Psychiatry 2003; 54:804–814.

6 Trivedi, MH, Rush AJ, Wisniewski SR, et al. Evaluation of outcomes with citalopram for depression. Using measurement-based care in STAR*D: implications for clinical practice. Am J Psychiatry 2006; 163:1–13.

7 Folstein MF, Folstein SE, McHugh PR. Mini-mental state. A practical method for grading the cognitive status of patients for the clinician. J Psychiatr Res 1975; 12:189–198.

# Chapter 4

# Principles of therapy

Ian M Anderson

The overriding principle behind the treatment of depression is to optimize treatment on an individual basis in order to meet the needs of the patient and to obtain the best possible clinical outcome. This involves not only careful assessment and application of the best evidence by the doctor or therapist but also sensitivity to the wishes, concerns, and beliefs of the patient. To be successful, treatment should be a mutual enterprise based on negotiation that recognizes the different roles of therapist and patient, and the patient's rights to make informed choices.

## Goals of treatment

In an obvious sense, the ultimate goal of treatment is straightforward – to return the sufferer from depression to a state of full health. However, it is important to recognize that this can be interpreted differently: the patient may have different expectations from the doctor or therapist, and goals may need to be tempered by practical considerations and unwanted effects of treatment.

Figure 4.1 shows some of the phase-specific outcomes that need to be considered. Traditionally, research and clinical practice have focused on acute phase symptomatic improvement, but other outcomes are equally important, especially to the depression sufferer, and include positive mental health such as optimism and self-confidence, a return to one's usual self, and a return to usual level of functioning [1].

The different outcomes tend to be highly correlated in uncomplicated depression, although functional improvement tends to lag behind symptomatic improvement. Factors other than depression impact on function and well-being, including medical and psychiatric comorbidity, and personality and social factors. However, depression has been shown to cause greater health decrements than other common chronic physical diseases [2], and effective treatment of comorbid depression can greatly improve quality of life.

E. Friedman and I.M. Anderson, *Managing Depression in Clinical Practice*
DOI 10.1007/978-1-84996-465-4_4, © Springer-Verlag London Limited 2010

| Treatment goals | | | |
|---|---|---|---|
| | | Assessment | |
| Outcomes | Acute phase | Continuation phase | Maintenance phase |
| Symptoms | Response<br>Remission | Stable remission | Stable recovery |
| Adverse effects | ← Good tolerability and safety → | | |
| Function | Improved social and occupational function | Regained full social and occupational function | Maintained full social and occupational function |
| Wellbeing | Improved quality of life | Regained quality of life | Maintained quality of life |

Figure 4.1 Treatment goals

It is increasingly that longer-term outcomes are just as important as acute treatment [3] and the goal of achieving stable remission/recovery and preventing relapse needs to be emphasized (see Chapter 8).

## Rating scales for assessment of outcomes

A variety of observer-rated and self-report measures are available to assess both severity and outcome after treatment and some of the most common are listed in Figure 4.2. Self-report measures have been seen as increasingly important but have not replaced observer-rated symptom measures as primary outcomes, especially in studies used to license drugs.

Quality of life is judged a subjective state and relies on self-report measures. Adverse effects, although very important for treatment adherence and quality of life, have received less systematic attention than efficacy outcomes.

## Acute treatment outcomes

Commonly reported symptomatic outcomes are:

- Response, usually defined as 50% or greater improvement in a rating scale score, especially Hamilton Depression Rating Scale (HDRS) or Montgomery Åsberg Depression Rating Scale (MADRS).
- Remission, absent or minimal depressive symptoms, usually defined as scoring below a cut-off on a rating scale. Accepted values are <8 on the 17-item HDRS and <10 (or sometimes <13) on the MADRS.

Partial remission is used to refer to patients who continue to have significant symptoms but are below the threshold for major depression and typically score between 8 and 13 on the 17-item HDRS. Full remission is associated with much better functional and quality-of-life outcomes compared with partial remission [5].

| Commonly used outcome measures | | |
|---|---|---|
| Outcome | Measure | Comment |
| Observer rated | | |
| Symptoms | Hamilton Depression Rating Scale (HDRS)<br>Montgomery–Åsberg Depression Rating Scale (MADRS)<br>Clinical Global Impression (CGI) | The HDRS has a greater emphasis on somatic symptoms compared with the MADRS. The CGI is a single overall assessment of illness severity |
| Adverse effects | Spontaneous report | Although categorization of AEs has been standardized, systematically elicited assessment is rare |
| Function | Global Assessment of Functioning (GAF) | GAF is a composite measure of symptom severity and function |
| Self-rated | | |
| Symptoms | Beck Depression Inventory (BDI)<br>Hospital Anxiety and Depression Scale (HADS)<br>Patient Health Questionnaire (PHQ-9)<br>Quick Inventory of Depressive Symptomatology – Self Rated (QIDS-SR) | BDI is widely used and covers the range of depressive symptoms<br>HADS includes anxiety assessment and omits somatic symptoms<br>PHQ-9 rates how often depressive symptoms have been present rather than severity<br>QIDS-SR – see Figure 3.2 |
| Adverse effects (AEs) | Global AE questionnaires not commonly used | Questionnaires for specific AEs are sometimes used (e.g., for sexual AEs) |
| Function | Medical Outcomes Study Short Form 36 (SF-36) | The SF-36 assesses functioning and health status |
| Quality of life | EQ-5D | A simple global health measure used for health economic analyses |

Figure 4.2 Commonly used outcome measures. Adapted from [4].

Figure 4.3 illustrates the relationship between response and remission. Although response is a useful measure, particularly when comparing treatments, there has been increasing emphasis on remission as the main outcome, because it relates better to the outcomes valued by depression sufferers: freedom from symptoms, and good function and wellbeing [1].

Figure 4.3 also illustrates that depression severity improves initially over time and then plateaus. The time frame of individual studies influences the proportion of patients who will achieve response and particularly remission in that study. There are no comparable agreed definitions for improvements in function or wellbeing measures.

**Relationship between response and remission over time depending on initial severity of depression**

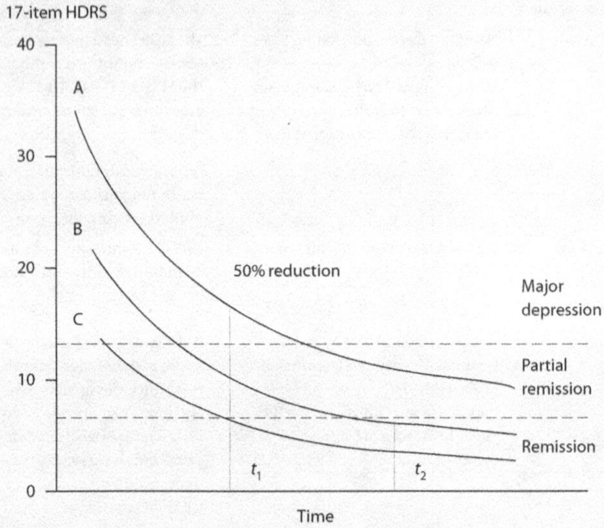


Figure 4.3 Relationship between response and remission over time depending on initial severity of depression. Patient A with severe depression still meets criteria for major depression at $t_1$ after improving sufficiently to have responded; by the end of the time period they are below the threshold for major depression but have still not fully remitted. Patient B with moderate depression responds and is in partial remission at $t_1$ but does not achieve remission until $t_2$. Patient C with mild depression meets criteria for both response and remission at $t_1$.

Although these definitions are useful there are inevitably patients whose treatment course does not fit this clear pattern and who either do not respond sufficiently to treatment (see Chapter 7) or have a fluctuating course with unstable response and/or remission.

## Medium- and long-term treatment outcomes

After the acute treatment phase with its aim of achieving full remission, there is a period of consolidation termed "continuation" treatment in order to prevent early worsening, or relapse. This has been defined in the context of patients taking antidepressants; there is less evidence about the early post-treatment period with psychological treatments, although a few booster or follow-up sessions are commonly offered. Consideration then needs to be given to whether ongoing "maintenance" or prophylactic treatment is required to prevent recurrence of a further depressive episode – see Chapter 8.

## Treatment options

### Nonspecific effects and placebo

One of the major problems in assessing the efficacy of treatments is the tendency for improvement to occur unrelated to specific aspects of treatment. This is best known in relation to the use of placebo tablets in drug trials but also applies to psychotherapies that posit a specific mechanism (e.g., CBT). Factors that are believed to contribute to response to placebo are given in Figure 4.4.

**Factors contributing to response to a placebo treatment in drug trials**

| Type | Examples |
|---|---|
| Illness factors | Spontaneous improvement |
| Measurement errors | Regression to the mean<br>Observer or patient biases |
| Placebo (nonspecific) effects | Expectation of benefit<br>Sharing of feelings, support, and structure<br>Engagement of coping mechanisms and empowerment<br>Behavioral change<br>Neural mechanisms, such as conditioning |

Figure 4.4 Factors contributing to response to a placebo treatment in drug trials

The placebo effect refers to the nonspecific, but genuinely beneficial, effects of engaging in a treatment. The degree of benefit and which factors contribute differ depending on the condition and the individual. Deliberately giving a placebo drug is unethical (outside a clinical trial with informed consent) and the effects are not consistent. Maximizing nonspecific beneficial effects is, however, an important (and large) part of the overall effect of treatment and should not be overlooked.

Spontaneous improvement and placebo effects are greatest in milder degrees of depression and smaller when the disorder is more severe and/or chronic. In the mildest degrees of depression, studies have shown response rates of 50–60% to placebo compared with less than 30% in moderate-to-severe depression [7–9].

### Specific treatment options

The main specific treatment options in clinical use are given in Figure 4.5. Details about the individual treatments are given in subsequent chapters.

## Choice of treatment

### Thresholds for benefit from specific treatments

An important decision is at what stage specific treatments (such as antidepressants or CBT) are needed when an individual presents with depression. This does not mean that people with mild depression do not require, or benefit from, help, but rather directs the clinician to the type of help that is appropriate.

Placebo-controlled drug studies and the rather fewer psychological treatment studies against active control conditions indicate that little is to be gained by specific treatment over nonspecific support in milder, shorter duration states of depression because people do equally well with both. The issue is, therefore, how to maximize benefit while minimizing unnecessary treatment – for reasons of both cost and potential harm (e.g., antidepressant adverse effects).

Severity and duration of depression are dimensions that have somewhat arbitrarily been divided into "categories" (e.g., minor depression, different severities of major depression). There is no "threshold" of clinical benefit from specific treatments over placebo; it increases as severity, and to some extent duration, increase (although this is probably not a linear effect).

**Types of treatment**

| Modality | Main groupings |
|---|---|
| Medications | Selective serotonin reuptake inhibitors<br>Serotonin and norepinephrine reuptake inhibitors<br>Tricyclic antidepressants<br>Norepinephrine reuptake inhibitors<br>Monoamine oxidase inhibitors<br>Others including receptor antagonists, such as trazodone and mirtazapine |
| Psychological treatments | Nondirective therapy/counseling<br>Directed self-help/computerized cognitive-behavioral therapy<br>Problem-solving therapy<br>Cognitive-behavioral therapy<br>Behavior therapy/behavioral activation<br>Interpersonal psychotherapy |
| Physical treatments | Electroconvulsive therapy<br>Bright light therapy<br>Experimental brain stimulation techniques |
| Other/complementary treatments | St John's wort<br>Omega-3-fatty acids<br>Folic acid |

Figure 4.5 Types of treatment

It is important to individually tailor treatment, bearing in mind the patient's illness history and preferences. Clinical judgment is called for rather than rigid rules in applying the evidence base to individuals [10].

Nevertheless current clinical "categories" do provide some indication of potential benefit for an "average" patient, so providing a starting point for treatment choice (Figure 4.2). The severity "threshold" of DSM-IV major depression appears to be where antidepressant benefits start to be detected, but this is only clearly clinically important at moderate severity or greater. This can be an issue for ICD-10-defined depression where the threshold for diagnosis of a depressive episode is lower than for DSM-IV (see Chapter 3), so that someone with mild ICD-10 depression may, on average, not routinely warrant specific treatment; with, for example, antidepressants.

By definition, 2 weeks is the minimum duration for major depression but little is known regarding how long it needs to have lasted before antidepressants have specific benefit. There is some evidence that spontaneous improvement is very common in the first 2 or 3 months [11], but in practice most patients will have had persisting symptoms before presenting for help. Minor depression (i.e., below the threshold for major depression) can be very disabling and, although structured supportive treatment should be considered initially, specific treatment is warranted if it persists (this includes dysthymia).

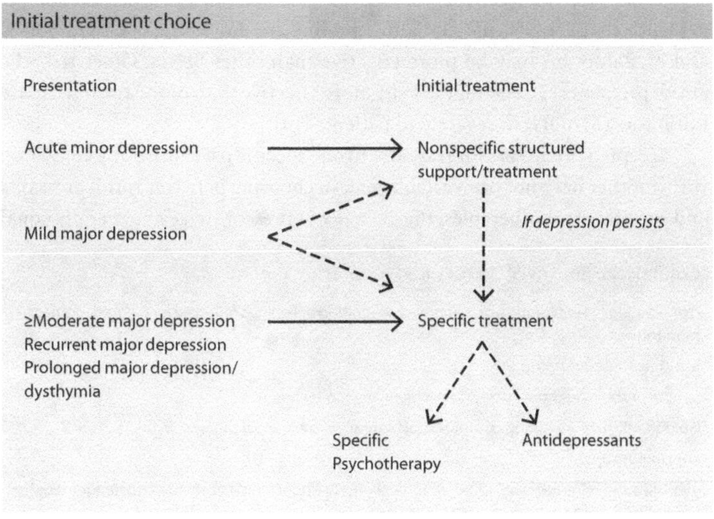


Figure 4.6 Initial treatment choice

The best way to deliver nonspecific structured support or treatment is not known and the term "watchful waiting" has been used. However, this can be taken to imply inaction, whereas limited evidence suggests that an active approach is needed to provide benefit. Figure 4.7 suggests some approaches to providing active nonspecific support.

## Choice between specific treatments

Unfortunately there is a lack of compelling evidence allowing confident prediction of who will respond to (or tolerate) one particular specific treatment better than another, be it an antidepressant or psychotherapy. The proposed predictors have included genetic markers (e.g., the serotonin transporter), gender, depression type, and comorbidities, but the evidence is generally conflicting. Some predictors are applied pragmatically (e.g., combining an antipsychotic with an antidepressant in psychotic depression, bright light therapy for seasonal affective disorder), but the others are of research interest or considered when initial treatment has failed [10].

There has been a great deal of interest in whether some antidepressants are more effective than others and how this relates to their pharmacology. It is generally accepted that any differences are marginal and that tolerability and side effects are the major factor in primary care. In more severe depression in secondary care, modest differences may be more important and there is some evidence that venlafaxine and amitriptyline are more effective than SSRIs, and escitalopram may be more effective than other SSRIs. Older tricyclic antidepressants (TCAs) may also be more effective than monoamine oxidase inhibitors (MAOIs) in severely ill patients [10].

Accepted predictors for response to one specific psychotherapy compared with another have not been established. In choosing between antidepressants and specific psychotherapies, the evidence at present suggests generally equal

| Examples of nonspecific structured support/treatment |
|---|
| Opportunity for exploration of issues and ventilation of feelings followed by defined regular monitoring |
| Nondirective counseling |
| Simple problem identification and problem-solving techniques |
| Guided self-help, including computerized cognitive–behavorial therapy |
| Support groups |
| Identification of regular social/recreational/exercise opportunities; provide encouragement, timetable and feedback progress at follow-up |

Figure 4.7 Examples of nonspecific structured support/treatment

acute efficacy, although chronically depressed patients with early childhood trauma may respond better to psychotherapy than to antidepressants. There is, however, a lack of evidence for psychological therapies in very severe depression and clinical observation is that such patients commonly lack the motivation and cognitive ability to engage in them. Combining antidepressants and psychotherapy from the start of treatment may give added benefit over either alone for more severely ill patients and for those with chronic depression, but not for those with mild-to-moderate depression. At the most severe end of the spectrum there is reasonable evidence that electroconvulsive therapy is the most effective treatment with significant acute benefit over medication [10].

## Practicalities of treatment

### Evaluation of risk, education, and agreeing treatment

Patients with depression can present a risk of suicide, occasionally harm to others (e.g., a depressed mother may kill her baby), or neglect. Severe depression and suicidality can make patients reject treatment or reduce their capacity so that informed treatment choice is not possible. In these cases, careful consideration has to be given to how and where treatment can be effectively and safely initiated (e.g., crisis intervention or in a hospital setting) and whether treatment needs to be given under Mental Health legislation. Most patients with mild-to-moderate depression are managed safely in primary care or outpatient settings.

An important and often overlooked aspect of managing depression is education. This consists of providing the patient with information about depression, in the context of their own history and experience. This requires the practitioner to understand depression and be able to evaluate the important factors in the patient's history. It is important in helping patients start to understand their illness and to engage nonspecific therapeutic factors (see above). It helps the therapeutic alliance and negotiation of, and engagement in, treatment. Often it can be helpful to enlist outside resources, the internet, written information, and voluntary organizations in the educational process.

It will be apparent that agreeing appropriate treatment requires evaluation of which treatments are indicated given the nature of the patient's illness (see Chapter 3), taking into account their individual characteristics, the availability of treatment, and their personal choice. This requires negotiation, with clinicians bringing their expertise and knowledge of depression, the benefits and risks of different treatments, and their availability to the situation. Patients bring their own beliefs, experience, and perceptions, which should be sensitively explored and, where necessary, misconceptions should be discussed. The aim is for patients to make an informed choice about treatment (within the bounds of what is possible). The negotiation and information given need to match the patient's wishes and ability, bearing in mind that the patient is in a vulnerable position, often desperate for help, and the depression may make absorbing and processing information difficult. It can be helpful to involve family members or care-givers in discussions, where necessary and with the patient's agreement. Figure 4.8 shows some general principles to apply in recommending particular treatments. Respecting patient choice as far as possible is very important in the therapeutic alliance and in achieving adherence to treatment, although there is surprisingly little evidence that this affects overall outcome.

| General principles in recommending treatments | |
|---|---|
| General | Take into account patient choice<br>Consider both short- and longer-term treatment needs<br>Prioritize treatments with a sound evidence base<br>Apply the principle of fully informed consent (requires discussion of alternative treatments, benefits, risks, off-label use of medication, etc)<br>Provide necessary education and information about what the patient can expect from treatment and any precautions to be taken<br>Consider practical availability of treatments |
| If medication is indicated | Match choice of antidepressant drug to individual patient requirements as far as possible<br>In principle choose antidepressants that are better tolerated and safer in overdose (older TCAs and MAOIs are second-line drugs)<br>Balance potential efficacy and adverse effects, according to patient needs |
| If specific psychotherapy is indicated | Prioritize treatments with an evidence base for depression, such as CBT, BT, and IPT<br>Recommend practitioners who have appropriate expertise/accreditation |

Figure 4.8 General principles in recommending treatments. BT, behavioral therapy; CBT, cognitive–behavioral therapy; IPT, interpersonal psychotherapy; MAOI, monoamine oxidase inhibitor; TCA, tricyclic antidepressant.

Figure 4.9 provides some considerations that may be helpful in recommending specific antidepressant treatments [10].

The choice between different psychotherapies has been relatively little studied and there is little evidence-based guidance possible. The therapist–patient relationship and therapist expertise (particularly in more severe depression) are fundamentally important and impact on the patient's engagement in therapy. In practice, choice is usually limited by what is available locally, particularly in a public health system.

| Choosing a specific antidepressant |
| --- |
| Previous history of treatment response, tolerability, and adverse effects to a particular antidepressant drug/drug class |
| Comorbid psychiatric disorder that may indicate a particular treatment (e.g., obsessive–compulsive disorder and SSRIs) |
| Likely side-effect profile |
| Low lethality in overdose if history or likelihood of overdose |
| Concurrent medical illness or condition that may make the antidepressant more noxious or less well tolerated |
| Concurrent medication that may interact with the antidepressant drug |
| Strong family history of differential antidepressant response |

Figure 4.9 Choosing a specific antidepressant. SSRI, selective serotonin reuptake inhibitor.

## Special populations

There are specific populations where special care or special considerations are needed.

### Children and adolescents

There is controversy about the use of antidepressants in younger age groups who are more likely to self-harm. The response to placebo treatment is high and appears to be responsible for the small antidepressant–placebo differences seen in adolescents and lack of clear efficacy in younger children [12]. There is also more concern that antidepressants may precipitate self-harm or suicidal behavior. For this reason there needs to be careful consideration about using antidepressants in this age group, with SSRIs being the best studied and the class with the best evidence base. TCAs and drugs more dangerous in overdose should be avoided where possible. Although psychological treatments are usually promoted as first-line treatment, it needs to be recognized that the evidence for the efficacy of specific psychotherapies over structured supportive care/treatment is not strong in this age group [10].

### Elderly people

The adage "start low and go slow" when prescribing medications to elderly people remains prudent advice. Medication for older adults is complicated by altered drug pharmacokinetics compared with younger adults, increased likelihood of drug–drug interactions (owing to increased medical comorbidity that results in use of multiple medications), and increased probability of adverse effects (such as orthostatic hypotension). Metabolism and clearance of metabolites are diminished in elderly people as a result of decreases in secretion in renal tubules, hepatic mass, and function of most of the cytochrome (CYP) enzymes. Decreases in albumin and other plasma proteins may impact on the protein binding of medications, further enhancing the sensitivity of older individuals to antidepressants [13].

The efficacy of antidepressants in the treatment of depression in elderly people has not been well established. A very limited literature of adequately powered, placebo-controlled studies reveals mixed results for fluoxetine, escitalopram, and venlafaxine; they all failed to demonstrate superiority to placebo in the treatment of geriatric patients with MDD, when using a 50% reduction in Hamilton Rating Scale for Depression (HAM-D) or MADRS score as a definition of response. This poor antidepressant response rate may reflect the predominance of several predictors of poor medication response: the presence of increased neurovegetative symptoms of depression, increased medical comorbidities, and increased medication intolerance. Interestingly, when the FDA reviewed suicidality and SSRIs across the lifespan, seeking to clarify risks that those agents might pose in younger people, patients aged 65 years and over displayed markedly reduced suicidal ideation and behavior (odds ratio 0.37 compared with placebo-treated patients) [14].

Psychotherapy for depression in elderly people has had many underpowered studies, and few comparing antidepressants with psychotherapy. Recently, paroxetine proved superior to placebo in maintenance treatment of depression in patients who had responded to the combination of paroxetine and interpersonal psychotherapy (IPT) acutely [15].

## Pregnancy and breastfeeding

Avoiding unnecessary medication in pregnancy is recommended, but, in general, TCAs and SSRIs have been used without evidence of significant adverse effects, although paroxetine is best avoided because of some concerns about cardiovascular defects. Third trimester antidepressants have been associated with a usually mild and self-limiting neonatal behavioral syndrome. Antidepressants vary in how much they are secreted in breast milk and citalopram and fluoxetine are best avoided if possible [10].

## Initiating treatment

When treatment is initiated it is important to provide information about what the patient can expect with treatment. It is well recognized that there is a delay between starting treatment and noticeable benefit, but contrary to standard teaching it does appear that improvement can be detected in the first few days and the greatest rate of benefit improvement, revealed by ratings of symptoms, occurs in the first 1 or 2 weeks. However, other aspects, such as function and sense of wellbeing, lag behind this so it is often 3 or 4 weeks before the patient feels any better. Improvement with psychological treatment tends to be a little slower. To gain the maximum benefit from antidepressants, always aim to treat at proven therapeutic doses.

The types of side effects that might occur with medication should be explained. Studies show that most patients experience some adverse effects early in treatment (although not all are directly due to the drug, as some occur with placebo treatment – see Chapter 5 for side effects from particular antidepressants). Most side effects are mild, occur in the first 2 weeks or so, and then improve. Emphasizing that the side effects will occur before benefit is experienced and will usually diminish is important in helping patients persevere with treatment. For some treatments (e.g., TCAs, reboxetine) it is helpful to titrate the dose up over about 1 or 2 weeks to minimize side effects. Other drugs (e.g., most SSRIs) are started at their therapeutic dose.

A controversy with antidepressants, especially SSRIs, concerns whether or not they might provoke suicidal thoughts or actions. Whether or not this might be the case for some vulnerable groups (e.g., adolescents and young adults), increased suicidality can occur during all types of treatment. Patients need to be warned that, if they experience increased agitation and/or suicidality, they should seek help immediately.

Patients often also stop treatment when they start to feel better. It is important to emphasize that antidepressant treatment needs to be continued after improvement in order to prevent early relapse, as there is a high risk of this in the months after remission. In addition, they need to be warned about the risk of a discontinuation reaction if antidepressants are stopped suddenly after treatment for more than a couple of months.

## Monitoring and adjusting treatment

Evidence shows that structured follow-up and monitoring are associated with better outcomes and even that the more frequent follow-up is better than less frequent. Early in treatment, it is advisable to make contact after 1 or 2 weeks to assess side effects and suicidality, and this can help patients to adhere to treatment.

Until recently it has been fairly rare in clinical practice to use standardized measures of mood assessment. On the analogy that a physician would not treat a patient with diabetes without measuring plasma glucose, it can be argued that simply using a global assessment of improvement is insufficient. Self-rated standardized assessments (see Figure 4.2) are easy to use and provide helpful symptom profile information (such as suicidality), as well as engaging patients in monitoring their own symptoms.

A systematic scheme of monitoring allows the application of so-called "critical decision points." These are specific points at which response to treatment is assessed and treatment changed if necessary. They have been used in medication treatment algorithms using standardized assessments and shown to produce benefit [16]. Figure 4.10 illustrates this. (See Chapter 7 for further discussion of treatment alteration for poor response.)

Critical decision points: guidelines in acute treatment with antidepressants

| Time (weeks) | Clinical assessment | Rating scale | Action |
|---|---|---|---|
| 4 | No improvement or worse | < 20% improvement | Consider altering treatment* |
| | Some improvement | > 20% improvement | Continue current treatment |
| 6 | Insufficient improvement | < 50% improvement | Consider altering treatment* |
| | Response | ≥ 50% improvement | Continue current treatment |
| 8–12 | Not in full remission | > Remission cut-off | Consider altering treatment* |
| | Full remission | < Remission cut-off | Continue current treatment for at least 4–6 months |

Figure 4.10 Critical decision points: guidelines in acute treatment with antidepressants. *Options include continuing current treatment if progress still being made, increasing dose, switching antidepressant, or adding in a second agent. For partial remission after 12 weeks consider adding CBT.

It is less clear how this model might apply to psychological treatments and it deserves study; for example, if insufficient improvement has occurred after four to six sessions, should alterations in treatment or adding medication be considered?

## Service structure in delivery of treatment

There is good evidence that the structure of treatment delivery is important in implementing the appropriate monitoring and adjustment of treatment. In primary care, collaborative care (broadly defined as structured care involving greater use of nonmedical specialists to augment treatment) and case management (continuity of care with at least systematic monitoring of symptoms) have been shown to lead to improved outcome compared with usual treatment; at least part of this appears to result from enhanced medication adherence [17]. The best way to enhance care is not known, but a minimum appears to be a structured system of follow-up (e.g., involving a case manager) and incorporating education about medication adherence.

In secondary care the structure of treatment has been less studied, but it does appear that using treatment algorithms and more intensive treatment regimens leads to better outcomes [18]. The National Institute for Health and Clinical Excellence (NICE) [19] outlined a stepped care approach to treatment, which provides a structure for matching patients to the appropriate service and type of treatment.

## Factors affecting response to treatment

Although most factors that might affect response cannot be changed, it is useful to consider their presence when planning treatment as some factors, such as adverse social conditions, may be amenable to intervention. Factors that are generally believed to be associated with poorer outcome of depression overall are earlier age of onset, duration and severity of depression, number of previous episodes, psychotic depression, failure of previous treatments, comorbidity with medical illness, anxiety disorders and substance misuse, some personality disorders, social factors such as ongoing social adversity, and cognitive impairment in elderly people [10,20,21].

When factors predicting response to antidepressant treatment in an episode of depression have been examined, fewer appear to influence outcome (Figure 4.11) [22]. What is important to take from this is that a range of interacting factors impacts on response to treatment, but it is difficult to predict from an individual factor what will happen in a particular patient.

There is less evidence with regard to response to treatment with psychological treatments, although one factor that came out strongly in a large study was large differences between individual therapists [23]. Although it has not been studied, it is also likely that there are clinician factors influencing response to antidepressant treatment given the large nonspecific component to treatment.

**Factors predicting response to antidepressant treatment**

| Not associated or inconsistent | Appears associated with poorer response |
|---|---|
| Age | Severity of illness (especially in first episode) |
| Gender | Comorbid anxiety |
| Age of onset | Poorer social support |
| Duration of episode | No partner/spouse |
| Number of recurrences | Unemployed, poorer education |
| | Significant physical illness |
| | Nonresponse to treatment in current episode |
| | Therapist factors |

Figure 4.11 Factors predicting response to antidepressant treatment

## References


1 Zimmerman M, McGlinchey JB, Posternak MA, et al. How should remission from depression be defined? The depressed patient's perspective. Am J Psychiatry 2006; 163:148–150.

2 Moussavi S, Chatterji S, Verdes E, et al. Depression, chronic diseases, and decrements in health: results from the World Health Surveys. Lancet 2007; 370:851–858.

3 Judd LL, Akiskal HS, Maser JD, et al. A prospective 12-year study of subsyndromal and syndromal depressive symptoms in unipolar major depressive disorders. Arch Gen Psychiatry 1998; 55:694–700.

4 Lam RW, Michalak EE, Swinson RP. Assessment Scales in Depression and Anxiety. London and New York: Taylor & Francis, 2005.

5 Meltzer-Brody S, Davidson JR. Completeness of response and quality of life in mood and anxiety disorders. Depress Anxiety 2000; 12(Suppl 1):95–101.

6 Guess HA, Kleinman A, Kusek JW, et al (eds). The Science of the Placebo: Towards an interdisciplinarly research agenda. London: BMJ Books, 2002.

7 Walsh BT, Seidman SN, Sysko R, et al. Placebo response in studies of major depression: variable, substantial, and growing. JAMA 2002; 287:1840–1847.

8 Angst J, Scheidegger P, Stabl M. Efficacy of moclobemide in different patient groups. Results of new subscales of the Hamilton Depression Rating Scale. Clin Neuropharmacol 1993; 16(Suppl 2):S55–S62.

9 Barrett JE, Williams JW Jr, Oxman TE, et al. Treatment of dysthymia and minor depression in primary care: a randomized trial in patients aged 18 to 59 years. J Fam Pract 2001; 50: 405–441.

10 Anderson I, Ferrier I, Baldwin R, et al. Evidence-based guidelines for treating depressive disorders with antidepressants: a revision of the 2000 British Association for Psychopharmacology guidelines. J Psychopharmacol 2008; 22:343–396.

11 Posternak MA, Solomon DA, Leon AC, et al. The naturalistic course of unipolar major depression in the absence of somatic therapy. J Nerv Ment Dis 2006; 194: 324–329.

12 Bridge JA, Iyengar S, Salary CB, et al. Clinical response and risk for reported suicidal ideation and suicide attempts in pediatric antidepressant treatment: a meta-analysis of randomized controlled trials. JAMA 2007; 297:1683–1696.

13 Lotrich F, Pollack B. Aging and clinical pharmacology: Implications for antidepressants. J Clin Pharmacol 2005; 45:1106–1122.

14 Food and Drug Administration. Clinical Review: Relationship between antidepressant drugs and suicidality in adults. Department of Health and Human Service, FDA, Center for Drug Evaluation and Research, 2006; 130:1.

15 Dombrovski A, Lentze E, Dew M, et al. Maintenance treatment for old-age depression preserves health-related quality of life: a randomized controlled trial of paroxetine and interpersonal therapy. J Am Geriatric Soc 2007; 55:1325–1332.

16 Adli M, Bauer M, Rush AJ. Algorithms and collaborative-care systems for depression: are they effective and why? A systematic review. Biol Psychiatry 2006; 59:1029–1038.

17 Gensichen J, Beyer M, Muth C. Case management to improve major depression in primary health care: a systematic review. Psychol Med 2006; 36: 7–14.

18 Trivedi MH, Rush AJ, Crismon ML, et al. Clinical results for patients with major depressive disorder in the Texas Medication Algorithm Project. Arch Gen Psychiatry 2004; 61: 669–680.

19 National Institute for Health and Clinical Excellence. Depression: the treatment and management of depression in adults. Clinical guideline 90, London: NICE, 2009. Accessible at http://guidance.nice.org.uk/CG90/NICEGuidance/pdf/English.

20 Meyers BS, Sirey JA, Bruce M, et al. Predictors of early recovery from major depression among persons admitted to community-based clinics: an observational study. Arch Gen Psychiatry 2002; 59:729–735.

21 Ezquiaga E, Garcia A, Bravo F, et al. Factors associated with outcome in major depression: a 6-month prospective study. Soc Psychiatry Psychiatr Epidemiol 1998; 33:552–557.

22 Bagby RM, Ryder AG, Cristi C. Psychosocial and clinical predictors of response to pharmacotherapy for depression. J Psychiatry Neurosci 2002; 27:250–257.
23 Okiishi JC, Lambert ML, Eggett E, et al. An analysis of therapist treatment effects: toward providing feedback to individual therapists on their clients' psychotherapy outcome. J Clin Psychol 2006; 62:1157–1172.

# Chapter 5

# Medications

Ian M Anderson and Danilo Arnone

The essence of the theoretical background of antidepressant action is based on the monoamine hypothesis of depression. In the 1960s, it was noted that reserpine, a catecholamine-depleting agent, induced depression and that this effect was reversed by antidepressants. The involvement of monoamines was also supported by the observations suggesting that dopamine (DA) and norepinephrine (noradrenaline; NE) were functionally deficient in depression and elevated in mania. Similarly, Ashcroft proposed that an indoleamine, now called serotonin (5-hydroxytryptamine; 5HT) was deficient in depression, leading eventually to the development of SSRIs. It is widely believed that the chronic administration of SSRIs resulting in 5HT reuptake blockade is responsible for the downregulation of $5HT_{1A}$-receptors present on the cell bodies of serotoninergic neurons. This effect reduces negative feedback, increasing 5HT neuronal firing and hence 5HT synaptic availability. This is a proposed mechanism to explain the delay between acute administration of an antidepressant and the therapeutic effect. It is unlikely to be the full explanation and does not generalize to drugs acting in different ways on the monoamine systems. It is also increasingly recognized that the onset of improvement with antidepressants is immediate, although significant clinical benefit takes some weeks to be evident. Current theories of the mechanism of action of antidepressants emphasize effects beyond the synapse such as neurotropic effects [1].

This chapter describes antidepressants prescribed in clinical practice, with tables for pharmacology and clinical details of compounds commonly used in day-to-day practice. For more detail readers are referred to textbooks of pharmacotherapy [1–3]. Dosage may vary according to clinical presentation and age group. Many compounds have recommended twice or even three times daily dosing based on the elimination half-life. However, in practice, antidepressants are often given once daily and there

E. Friedman and I.M. Anderson, *Managing Depression in Clinical Practice* 
DOI 10.1007/978-1-84996-465-4_5, 

is no evidence of benefit in giving any antidepressant more than once daily, except to reduce side effects by influencing peak plasma effects. More than once-daily administration may impair adherence, and for many drugs single night-time administration is acceptable and tolerable [4,5]. Average dose ranges are given, but these should be taken as guidelines only and reference to manufacturer's information and/or national formulary is advisable at the time of prescribing [6,7].

## Selective serotonin reuptake inhibitors

Most guidelines support the use of SSRIs as first-line pharmacological treatment for depression on the basis of their safety and tolerability. The principal mechanism of action of SSRIs is to inhibit the reuptake of 5HT into the presynaptic nerve terminal. In terms of toxicity in overdose, SSRIs are generally considered at low risk, especially if taken alone. The smallest dose likely to cause death is not clearly defined but believed to be around 1 g or 2 g. Differences in SSRI tolerability probably result largely from pharmacokinetic considerations but there are also subtle pharmacodynamic differences, with fluoxetine being the least selective for 5HT over NE, and sertraline having some DA reuptake at higher doses. Fluvoxamine appears least well tolerated, at least in doses >100 mg, but may be the least likely to cause sexual dysfunction, whereas paroxetine is the most likely. Paroxetine appears the most likely to cause discontinuation symptoms, and fluoxetine the least [8]. The pharmacology and clinical use of SSRIs are summarized in Figures 5.1 and 5.2.

**Pharmacology of SSRIs**

| Drug | Active metabolite | $t_{1/2}$ ($t_{1/2}$ of metabolite) | Metabolism | Hepatic enzyme inhibition |
|---|---|---|---|---|
| Citalopram | Negligible | 36 | Hepatic | Negligible |
| Escitalopram (*S*-enantiomer of citalopram) | Negligible | 36 | Hepatic | Negligible |
| Fluoxetine | Norfluoxetine | 72 (200) | Hepatic | CYP2D6, 3A4, 2C19 |
| Fluvoxamine | Negligible | 25 | Hepatic | CYP1A2 |
| Paroxetine | Negligible | 20 | Hepatic | CYP2D6, 2C9 |
| Sertraline | Desmethylsertraline | 25 (66) | Hepatic | CYP2D6 (weak) |

Figure 5.1 Pharmacology of SSRIs. $t_{1/2}$, half-life (in hours); CYP, cytochrome P450; SSRI, selective serotonin reuptake inhibitor.

| Clinical use of SSRIs | | | |
|---|---|---|---|
| **Medication** | **Usual daily dose (mg)** | **Main side effects** | **Significant interactions** |
| Citalopram | 20–40 | Nausea/vomiting, agitation, akathisia, insomnia/sedation, sexual dysfunction, dizziness, convulsions (rare), increased risk of suicidality (<30 years), hyponatremia (especially in the elderly), increased risk of bleeding, discontinuation syndrome. | MAOIs (serotonin syndrome)<br>Lithium (therapeutic, serotonin syndrome)<br>L-Tryptophan (therapeutic, serotonin syndrome)<br>St John's wort (serotonin syndrome) |
| Escitalopram (*S*-enantiomer of citalopram) | 10–20 | As for citalopram | As for citalopram |
| Fluoxetine | 20–40 | As for citalopram but insomnia and agitation more common, discontinuation syndrome less common | As for citalopram plus:<br>Antipsychotics (increased concentration)<br>Opiates (increased concentration)<br>TCAs (increased concentration) |
| Sertraline | 50–200 | As for citalopram | As for citalopram |
| Paroxetine | 20–40 | As for citalopram but discontinuation syndrome more common (slow discontinuation advisable) | As for fluoxetine |
| Fluvoxamine | 100–200 | As for citalopram but nausea more common | As for citalopram plus:<br>Some TCAs (increased concentration)<br>Olanzapine, clozapine (increased concentration)<br>Warfarin (increased concentration)<br>Propranolol (increased concentration) |

Figure 5.2 Clinical use of SSRIs. MAOI, monoamine oxidase inhibitor; SSRI, selective serotonin reuptake inhibitor; TCA, tricyclic antidepressant.

## Serotonin and norepinephrine reuptake inhibitors

Venlafaxine, duloxetine and milnacipran (licensed in France and Japan) are known as "dual action" reuptake inhibitors because of their action as selective 5HT and NE reuptake inhibitors. The pharmacology and clinical use of SNRIs are summarized in Figures 5.3 and 5.4.

**Pharmacology of SNRIs**

| Drug | Active metabolite | $t_{1/2}$ ($t_{1/2}$ of metabolite) | Metabolism | Hepatic enzyme inhibition |
|---|---|---|---|---|
| Venlafaxine | *O*-Desmethylvenlafaxine | 5 (11) | Hepatic | Negligible |
| Duloxetine | Negligible | 12 | Hepatic | CYP2D6, CYP1A2 |
| Milnacipram | Negligible | 8 | Negligible | Negligible |

Figure 5.3 Pharmacology of SNRIs. $t_{1/2}$, half-life (in hours); CYP, cytochrome P450; SNRI, selective norepinephrine reuptake inhibitor.

**Clinical use of SNRIs**

| Medication | Usual daily dose (mg) | Main side effects | Significant interactions |
|---|---|---|---|
| Venlafaxine | 75–225 XL<br>75– 375 | Nausea, insomnia, dry mouth, sedation, dizziness, sweating nervousness, headache, sexual dysfunction, hypertension at higher doses | MAOIs (serotonin syndrome)<br>Lithium (therapeutic, serotonin syndrome)<br>L-Tryptophan (therapeutic, serotonin syndrome)<br>St John's wort (serotonin syndrome) |
| Duloxetine | 60–120 | Nausea, insomnia, dizziness, dry mouth, constipation, anorexia, and increased blood pressure and heart rate | As venlafaxine plus<br>TCAs (increase concentration)<br>Antipsychotics (increase concentration)<br>May cause liver damage or exacerbate pre-existing liver damage (avoid alcohol) |
| Milnacipran | 100 | Nausea, vertigo, increased anxiety, sweats, shivering, dysuria, itching and testicle pain | As venlafaxine |

Figure 5.4 Clinical use of SNRIs. MAOI, monoamine oxidase inhibitor; SSRI, selective serotonin reuptake inhibitor; TCA, tricyclic antidepressant.

### Venlafaxine

The efficacy of venlafaxine is similar to TCAs (e.g., amitriptyline, clomipramine, and imipramine), but better tolerated. There is some evidence that its dual mechanism of action makes venlafaxine more efficacious in the treatment of more severe depressive disorders, and guidelines tend to favor its use in cases of lack of, or insufficient response to, SSRIs. However, dual action is believed to occur only at higher doses. Reuptake of 5HT occurs at a dose of 75 mg, whereas for blockade of NE, reuptake dose is 150 mg/day and greater. At the highest doses, venlafaxine may also be a DA reuptake inhibitor; it is contraindicated in patients at high risk of serious cardiac ventricular arrhythmia and uncontrolled hypertension. It is considered good practice to ensure that the patient is normotensive at the time of prescribing and to monitor blood pressure at doses of 300 mg/day or above. It is advisable to seek specialist supervision in case of doses reaching 300 mg/day and above.

### Duloxetine

Duloxetine is a 5HT and NE reuptake inhibitor with weak inhibition of DA reuptake. As part of its marketing it has been proposed as being particularly effective for painful physical symptoms occurring in depression but direct, evidence of this is lacking. Usual dosage is in the range of 60–120 mg/day. Although the starting dose is recommended as 60 mg, it is better to titrate up from 30 mg in antidepressant-naïve patients to improve tolerability.

### Milnacipran

Milnacipran is a dual reuptake inhibitor with slightly more action on NE reuptake. Metabolism does not involve the CYP450 system, and it is excreted as a mixture of active and inactivated compound. Renal, but not hepatic, disease delays excretion.

## Monoamine receptor antagonist drugs

The pharmacology and clinical use of monoamine receptor antagonist drugs are summarized in Figures 5.5 and 5.6.

### Trazodone and nefazodone

Trazodone is a $5HT_2$ antagonist and a mild 5HT reuptake inhibitor. Other pharmacological actions include NE and $\alpha_1$ antagonism and antihistamine properties. One of the major advantages of both trazodone and nefazodone is that they do not interfere with sexual function significantly, and both are metabolized by the liver. Nefazodone was withdrawn from the European market in 2003 due to hepatotoxicity. The use of nefazodone is subject to monitoring of hepatic function in the USA.

| Pharmacology of monoamine receptor antagonist drugs | | | | |
|---|---|---|---|---|
| Drug | Active metabolites | $t_{1/2}$ ($t_{1/2}$ of metabolite) | Metabolism | Hepatic enzyme inhibition |
| Trazodone | *m*-Chlorophenylpiperazine | 3–9 (up to 72) | Hepatic | Negligible |
| Nefazodone | Negligible | 2–4 | Hepatic | CYP3A4 |
| Mirtazapine | Negligible | 26–37 | Hepatic | Negligible |

Figure 5.5 Pharmacology of monoamine receptor antagonist drugs. $t_{1/2}$, half-life (in hours).

| Clinical use of monoamine receptor antagonist drugs | | | |
|---|---|---|---|
| Medication | Usual daily dose (mg) | Main side effects | Significant interactions |
| Trazodone | 150–300 | Sedation, dizziness, headache, nausea/ vomiting, tremor, postural hypotension, tachycardia, rarely priapism | Negligible |
| Nefazodone | 300–600 | As above apart from priapism; less sedative | TCAs (increased concentration)<br>Alprazolam (increased concentration)<br>Potentional hepatoxicity; its use is subject to monitoring of hepatic function in the USA |
| Mirtazapine | 15–45 | Increased appetite, weight gain, drowsiness, edema, dizziness, headache | Negligible |

Figure 5.6 Clinical use of monoamine receptor antagonist drugs. Mianserin is similar to mirtazapine but also antagonizes 1-presynaptic receptors, which decreases presynaptic stimulation of 5HT neurons. It has similar side effects to mirtazapine but is also associated with blood dyscrasias and complete blood count monitoring is required. CYP, cytochrome P450.

## Mirtazapine

Mirtazapine mechanisms of action include antagonism of $\alpha_2$-presynaptic receptors, which ultimately increases both NE and 5HT neurotransmission by increased cell firing and synaptic release; antagonism of postsynaptic $5HT_2$ and $5HT_3$ receptors, which may also improve the tolerability of mirtazapine but contribute to weight gain; and a potent antihistaminergic effect contributing to its side effects of weight gain, sedation, and anxiolytic properties.

Mianserin is similar to mirtazapine but also antagonizes $\alpha_1$-presynaptic receptors, which decreases presynaptic stimulation of 5HT neurons. It has similar side effects to mirtazapine but is also associated with blood dyscrasias and complete blood count monitoring is required.

## Norepinephrine reuptake inhibitors

### Reboxetine

Reboxetine is a specific reuptake inhibitor of NE. Dosage is usually between 8 and 12 mg/day in twice-daily administration. Side effects include insomnia, sweating, dizziness, dry mouth, constipation, tachycardia, urinary retention, and sexual dysfunction. Dose titration may improve its tolerability. The pharmacology and clinical use of reboxetine is summarized in Figures 5.7 and 5.8.

**Pharmacology of reboxetine**

| Drug | Active metabolites | $t_{1/2}$ ($t_{1/2}$ of metabolite) | Metabolism | Hepatic enzyme inhibition |
|---|---|---|---|---|
| Reboxetine | Negligible | 13 | Hepatic | CYP3A4 inhibitor (e.g., erythromycin, ketoconazole) may increase its plasma concentration |

Figure 5.7 Pharmacology of reboxetine. $t_{1/2}$, half-life (in hours); CYP, cytochrome P450.

**Clinical use of reboxetine**

| Medication | Usual daily dose (mg) | Main side effects | Significant interactions |
|---|---|---|---|
| Reboxetine | 8–12 | Insomnia, sweating, dizziness, dry mouth, constipation, tachycardia, urinary retention, sexual dysfunction | Potentiation of benzodiazepine effect (↓ excretion) |

Figure 5.8 Clinical use of reboxetine

## Dopamine reuptake inhibitors

### Bupropion (amfebutamone)

The mechanism of action of bupropion is not fully understood but the main action is thought to be the inhibition of DA reuptake, although it is also a mild NE reuptake inhibitor. Bupropion is licensed in the USA for the treatment of depression, but in the UK it is licensed as a smoking cessation compound. It is available in immediate-release and two different delayed-release forms. Its use includes augmentation with SSRIs for treatment-resistant depression. At high doses it may cause seizures and it is contraindicated in cases of history of, or susceptibility to, developing seizures. Its metabolism mainly involves CYP2D6. The pharmacology and clinical use of buproprion is summarized in Figures 5.9 and 5.10.

| Pharmacology of bupropion | | | | |
|---|---|---|---|---|
| Drug | Active metabolites | $t_{1/2}$ ($t_{1/2}$ of metabolite) | Metabolism | Hepatic enzyme inhibition |
| Bupropion (amfebutamone) | *R,R*-Hydroxybupropion, *S,S*-Hydroxybupropion, *threo*-Hydrobupropion, *erythro*-Hydrobupropion | 10 (up to 26) | Hepatic | Hydroxybupropion CYP2D6 inhibitor |

Figure 5.9 Pharmacology of bupropion. $t_{1/2}$, half-life (in hours); CYP, cytochrome P450.

| Clinical use of bupropion | | | |
|---|---|---|---|
| Medication | Usual daily dose (mg) | Main side effects | Significant interactions |
| Bupropion (amfebutamone) | 300–450 | Dry mouth, insomnia, anxiety, gastrointestinal disturbance, sweating and hypertension | MAOIs (serotonin syndrome)<br>Carbamazepine/phenytoin (reduced concentration of bupropion)<br>Valproate (increased concentration bupropion)<br>Citalopram (increased concentration of citalopram) |

Figure 5.10 Clinical use of bupropion. MAOI, monoamine oxidase inhibitor.

## Tricyclic antidepressants

TCAs are amines that inhibit the reuptake of 5HT and NE. Tertiary amines (amitriptyline, imipramine, and clomipramine) are more potent 5HT blockers, whereas secondary amines (nortriptyline, desipramine, protriptyline) are more effective on NE. Other effects are anticholinergic and antihistaminergic. Tertiary amines are metabolized to secondary amines; for example, amitriptyline to nortriptyline, imipramine to desmethylimipramine (desipramine). Desipramine has been largely superseded by more modern compounds but is still available in the USA. TCAs have high toxicity and fatality in overdose, particularly dosulepin, amitriptyline, and desipramine. Amitriptyline and desipramine should be prescribed with caution in cases of high suicide risk (e.g., limited prescription, supervised administration) and dosulepin avoided. Lofepramine is the least toxic of all TCAs and clomipramine intermediate. The pharmacology and clinical use of TCAs are summarized in Figures 5.11 and 5.12.

## Pharmacology of TCAs

| Drug | $t_{1/2}$ ($t_{1/2}$ of metabolite) | Metabolism | Comparative pharmacology | | | |
|---|---|---|---|---|---|---|
| | | | NE reuptake inhibition | 5HT reuptake inhibition | Anticho-linergic effects | Sedation |
| Amitriptyline | 16 (36) | Hepatic | ++ | +++ | +++ | +++ |
| Imipramine | 16 (24) | Hepatic | ++ | +++ | ++ | ++ |
| Clomipramine | 18 (36) | Hepatic | + | +++ | +++ | + |
| Nortriptyline | 36 | Hepatic | +++ | + | ++ | + |
| Dosulepin (dothiepin) | 20 (40) | Hepatic | + | + | ++ | ++ |
| Lofepramine | 5 (24) | Hepatic | +++ | + | + | + |

Figure 5.11 Pharmacology of TCAs. *5HT, 5-hydroxytryptamine; CYP, cytochrome P450; NE, noradrenaline; TCA, tricyclic antidepressant;* $t_{1/2}$, *half-life (in hours).*

## Clinical use of TCAs

| Medication | Usual daily dose (mg) | Main side effects | Significant interactions |
|---|---|---|---|
| Amitriptyline | 75–150* | Dry mouth, blurred vision, constipation, urinary retention, sedation, postural hypotension, tachycardia/arrhythmia, weight gain | MAOIs (toxicity)<br>Paroxetine, fluoxetine (↑ levels of TCAs)<br>Phenothiazines (↑ levels of TCAs)<br>Cimetidine (↑ levels of TCAs)<br>Antimuscarinics (enhanced effect)<br>Alcohol |
| Imipramine | 75–150* | As for amitriptyline but less sedative | As for amitriptyline<br>MAOIs (toxicity, serotonin syndrome) |
| Clomipramine | 75–150* | As for amitriptyline | As for amitriptyline (but less sedating) except<br>MAOIs (toxicity marked) |
| Nortriptyline | 50–150 | As for amitriptyline but less sedative, anticholinergic and hypotensive. Constipation is common | As for amitriptyline |
| Dothepin (dosulepin)† | 75–225 | As for amitriptyline | As for amitriptyline |
| Lofepramine† | 140–210 | As for amitriptyline but less sedative, anticholinergic and hypotensive and low cardiotoxicity. Sweating | As for amitriptyline |

Figure 5.12 Clinical use of TCAs. *Higher doses (e.g., up to 200–300 mg are commonly used in the USA). †Not available in the USA. MAOI, monoamine oxidase inhibitor; TCA, tricyclic antidepressant.

**Pharmacology of MAOIs**

| Drug | $t_{1/2}$ ($t_{1/2}$ of metabolite) | Metabolism | Comparative pharmacology |
|---|---|---|---|
| Moclobemide | 2–4 | Hepatic | Reversible inhibitor of MAO-A |
| Phenelzine | 1.5 | Hepatic | Irreversible, nonselective MAO-A and -B inhibitor |
| Tranylcypromine | 2.5 | Hepatic | Irreversible, nonselective MAO-A and -B inhibitor |
| Isocarboxazid | 36 | Hepatic | Irreversible, nonselective MAO-A and -B inhibitor |
| Selegiline | 2 | Hepatic* | Irreversible, MAO-B > MAO-A inhibitor |

Figure 5.13 Pharmacology of MAOIs. $t_{1/2}$, half-life (in hours); CYP, cytochrome P450; MAOI, monoamine oxidase inhibitor. *First-pass metabolism reduced by administration as transdermal patch.

**Clinical use of MAOIs**

| Medication | Usual daily dose (mg) | Main side effects | Significant interactions |
|---|---|---|---|
| Moclobemide | 150–600 | Sleep disturbance, headache, nausea, agitation | Other antidepressants, pethidine, alcohol, barbiturates, insulin |
| Phenelzine | 45–60 | Postural hypotension, dizziness, drowsiness, insomnia, headaches, edema, anticholinergic effects, weight gain, restlessness, sexual difficulties, sweating, tremor | Tyramine in food, sympathomimetics, alcohol, opioids, other antidepressants, L-dopa |
| Tranylcypromine | 20–30 | As for phenelzine. More stimulating than phenelzine | As for phenelzine but interactions more severe and it is not advisable to use in combination |
| Isocarboxazid | 10–40 | As for phenelzine | Tyramine in food, sympathomimetics, alcohol, opioids, other antidepressants, L-dopa |
| Selegiline† | 6–12* | Headaches, diarrhoea, insomnia, skin reaction | Sympathomimetics, opioids, carbamazepine, other antidepressants |

Figure 5.14 Clinical use of MAOIs. MAOI, monoamine oxidase inhibitor. *Administration as transdermal patch. †Not available in Europe

## Monoamine oxidase inhibitors

MAOIs are inhibitors of MAO enzymes A and B. These enzymes are widely distributed in the CNS, but also peripherally, especially in the gastrointestinal system. MAO-A metabolizes NE, 5HT, DA, and tyramine, whereas the substrates of MAO-B are DA, tyramine, and phenylethylamine.

The inhibitory action of MAOIs results in an increased availability (storage and release) of 5HT and NE. Lack of selectivity for the CNS and irreversibility of the inhibition (for older compounds) are responsible for the most significant side effects. The most dangerous phenomenon associated with MAOIs is a hypertensive "cheese reaction" attributable to tyramine-containing foods (e.g., cheese, yeast extracts, hung game, some alcoholic drinks, broad bean pods, pickled herring), normally inactivated in the gut by MAO. Another cause is related to indirect sympathomimetic drugs such as phenylephrine (e.g., nonprescription cold remedies).

Symptoms include flushing, headache, increased blood pressure, cerebrovascular accident. The most effective treatment of this condition is $\alpha$-adrenergic blockade with phentolamine or chlorpromazine. MAOIs are generally contraindicated in cardio- and cerebrovascular disease, children, epilepsy, hepatic disease, pheocromocytoma, and hyperthyroidism. Irreversible MAOIs include traditional molecules (phenelzine, isocarboxazid, tranylcypromine) and selective MAO-B inhibitors (e.g., selegiline). Selegiline transdermal patches have been licensed in the USA for the treatment of depression. This reduces first-pass metabolism and the risk of hypertensive reactions and food restrictions. The only available reversible MAOI is moclobemide, an MAO-A inhibitor, also called a RIMA (reversible inhibitor of MAO-A). At usual doses moclobemide does not necessitate dietary restrictions as competitive antagonism allows tyramine to displace moclobemide from MAO.

As a result of the risk of adverse reactions, the traditional MAOIs should be reserved for patients failing other antidepressants and prescribed under specialist supervision.

The pharmacology and clinical use of MAOIs are summarized in Figures 5.13 and 5.14.

## Other drugs

### New compounds

Agomelatine was licensed in Europe at the end of 2008, subject to liver function test monitoring. Its chemical structure is closely related to melatonin, and it is an agonist at melatonin receptors and antagonist at $5HT_{2C}$-receptors. Agomelatine appears to have a benign side-effect profile and to help sleep. O-Desmethylvenlafaxine, which is currently in the prelicensing phase, is the principal metabolite of venlafaxine with a similar pharmacology. It is not clear what advantages it has over the parent compound.

### Augmentation strategies

Augmentation strategies include synergistic prescribing of antidepressants and/or other compounds including lithium, $T_3$, and atypical antipsychotics. Chapter 6 describes the use of augmentation strategies as next-step treatments. Their use should be supervised by mental health specialists. The clinical use of lithium is further described but for other drugs the reader is referred to the appropriate reference book, such as the *British National Formulary* (BNF) [6].

Lithium (usually given as lithium carbonate) is the best-established augmentation treatment, but its popularity has decreased with the availability of new drugs and the complexities of its use. It has multiple potential actions including enhancing 5HT function. It has a narrow therapeutic range and needs regular blood tests to maintain a serum concentration in the range of 0.5–1.0 mmol/L (preferably <0.8 mmol/L to minimize side effects). Lithium is excreted by the kidneys and can interfere with thyroid hormone release and affect cardiac conduction. Pre-treatment assessment of renal and thyroid function is required and, if indicated, cardiovascular status including an EKG (ECG). Monitoring of renal and thyroid function is required approximately every 6 months. Adverse effects include polyuria and polydipsia, tremor, gastrointestinal symptoms, and a metallic taste in the mouth. Dehydration, sodium depletion (diarrhea, sweating), hypovolemia, and renal failure can increase serum lithium concentrations leading to lithium toxicity, which requires immediately stopping lithium, and medical assessment and intervention, including dialysis, if levels are very high.

## Specific adverse effects of antidepressants

### Serotonin syndrome

The serotonin syndrome is an acute neuropsychiatric condition due to increased CNS 5HT activity. Rarely, it can be an idiosyncratic reaction to a serotoninergic drug but usually it results from a pharmacodynamic interaction between drugs that enhance 5HT function (e.g., SSRI + MAOI). Symptoms include confusion, myoclonic jerks, hyperreflexia, pyrexia, sweating, autonomic instability, gastrointestinal symptoms, mood change, and mania. Management is based on stopping the offending drug(s) and supportive measures [9].

### Antidepressant discontinuation syndrome

The discontinuation syndrome usually occurs only after antidepressant treatment has been established for some weeks and occurs on stopping the drug, especially if it is done abruptly, with symptoms starting in the first few days. The symptoms are variable and differ between classes of antidepressants but include sleep disturbance, gastrointestinal symptoms, affective symptoms, and general somatic symptoms such as lethargy and headache. In addition, SSRIs are associated with sensory symptoms, such as electric shock feelings and paraesthesia, and disequilibrium symptoms. MAOIs may cause more severe symptoms, including worsening depression and anxiety, confusion, and psychotic symptoms. With most antidepressants, psychotic symptoms, mania, and extrapyramidal symptoms have rarely been reported. Paroxetine and venlafaxine have been associated with high rates of discontinuation symptoms, whereas fluoxetine appears to have low rates, presumably due to its long half-life.

Management is based on education and reassurance, which suffice in most cases because the course tends to be mild and self-limiting (1 or 2 weeks). In more severe cases the implicated medication can be restarted and tapered more slowly. For SSRIs and SNRIs, fluoxetine can be prescribed and then stopped because its long half-life produces a natural taper. Prevention of the discontinuation syndrome can usually be achieved by tapering down the antidepressant dose over a few weeks.

### Suicidality

There has been recent concern that some antidepressants, particularly SSRIs, might cause increased suicidality in some patients. However, the evidence considered overall does not support an increased risk of completed suicide or clinically significant increased risk of suicidal behavior in adults with antidepressant use, and population studies have tended to find that antidepressants are associated with decreased suicide rates. However, individual sensitivity cannot be ruled out and SSRIs may be associated with a very small increase in nonfatal suicidal ideation/behavior in adolescents. More important is the recognition that all patients can experience an increase in suicidality during treatment and that this needs appropriate management (see Chapter 4) [10].

## References


1 Anderson IM, Reid IC (eds). Fundamentals of Clinical Psychopharmacology, 3rd edition. London: Informa UK Ltd, 2006.
2 Stahl SM. Essential Psychopharmacology. Cambridge: Cambridge University Press, 2006.
3 Shiloh R, Stryjer R, Nutt DJ (eds). Atlas of Psychiatric Pharmacotherapy, 2nd edition. London: Informa Healthcare, 2005.
4 Yildiz A, Pauler DK, Sachs GS. Rates of study completion with single versus split daily dosing of antidepressants: a meta-analysis. J Affect Disord 2004; 78:157–162.
5 Yyldyz A, Sachs GS. Administration of antidepressants. Single versus split dosing: a meta-analysis. J Affect Disord 2001; 66:199–206.
6 British National Formulary. London: BMJ Publishing Group Ltd and RPS Publishing, 2008.
7 Taylor D, Paton C, Kerwin R (eds). The Maudsley Prescribing Guidelines, 9th edition. London: Informa Healthcare, 2007.
8 Edwards JG, Anderson I. Systematic review and guide to selection of selective serotonin reuptake inhibitors. Drugs 1999; 57:507–533.
9 Haddad P, Dursan S, Deakin W (eds). Adverse syndromes and psychiatric drugs: a clinical guide. New York: Oxford University Press, 2004.
10 Anderson I, Ferrier I, Baldwin R, et al. Evidence-based guidelines for treating depressive disorders with antidepressants: a revision of the 2000 British Association for Psychopharmacology guidelines. J Psychopharmacol 2008; 22:343–396.

# Chapter 6

# Other treatments

Edward S Friedman

## Psychotherapy for depression

Several depression-focused psychotherapies [1] have been developed to be time-limited treatments. They have an explicit goal of helping the individual achieve rapid relief of depressive symptoms, inasmuch as they are treatments comparable to pharmacotherapy in time course and efficacy. Furthermore, by emphasizing short-term goals, these therapies capitalize on the acute nature of many episodes of depression. Shared features of the depression-focused psychotherapies include their specific linkage of a theoretical model of phenomenology with strategies for symptom reduction, with specification of methods to facilitate training and enhance fidelity, and with acceptance of the need to identify observable and measurable goals and outcomes. The major types of time-limited depression-focused therapies that have reliably established comparability to antidepressant medications in RCTs include cognitive therapy (CBT) [2] and IPT [3]. The particular theoretical orientation of each model of treatment also yields predictions about specific outcomes, such as the effects of CBT on measures of dysfunctional attitudes or IPT on measures of social adjustment. Finally, these therapies share several pragmatic features, including their compatibility for use in combination with pharmacotherapy and their suitability for use by therapists with a range of backgrounds and training.

IPT aims to relieve depression through the recognition that depression occurs within an interpersonal context regardless of its severity, phenomenology, or presumed etiology. IPT therapists help patients to understand and modify interpersonal problems associated with depression. Additional long-term benefits include improved social function and prophylaxis against relapse. IPT developed from the recognition that high rates of life stressors are associated with the onset of unipolar depression. Consequently, IPT often focuses on the relationship between attachment bonds and vulnerability to

E. Friedman and I.M. Anderson, *Managing Depression in Clinical Practice* 
DOI 10.1007/978-1-84996-465-4_6, 

depression. Helping the patient strengthen his or her intimate relationships may enhance the apparent protective or "neutralizing" role of social support. Another important aspect of the depressed person's social milieu is his or her performance in the workplace, with friends and peer groups, and in the neighborhood or community. Attention to social role performance thus includes the individual's current and long-term patterns of functioning in diverse situations, as well as more recent or still-evolving role transitions. IPT is a psychoeducational intervention because, in addition to the strong social emphasis, therapists teach patients about depression and its treatment. This includes providing practical advice or recommendations to help patients better tolerate the symptoms of depression and manage impairments associated with the depressive state. These efforts also serve to help lessen the demoralization and hopelessness experienced by most depressed people. The therapy may be quite active in this regard, including providing assistance to patients through the use of problem-solving strategies. IPT therapists are encouraged to identify one or more of four common interpersonal conflict situations to serve as the focus for therapeutic change: unresolved grief, role disputes, role transitions, and interpersonal deficits.

The cognitive model of depression and CBT derive from the work of Aaron Beck [2]. Beck recognized that depressed patients view themselves, the world, and their future in a negative manner (*the cognitive triad*). These negative cognitions (*automatic negative thoughts*) provide the gateway for the cognitive therapist to understand the depressed patient's phenomenological world. The patient is taught to identify and challenge dysfunctional thoughts, understand their guiding beliefs, and revise their dysfunctional attitudes. Therapists help patients discover their unconscious attitudes through the use of Socratic questioning and guided discovery exercises. According to the CBT model, depression results from unconscious dysfunctional beliefs being activated by current environmental stimuli, eliciting thoughts of helplessness, hopelessness, and worthlessness. It is believed that adverse early experiences are responsible for the individual learning inadequate coping strategies. This stress–diathesis model may explain why only some individuals become depressed after a stressor such as divorce or unemployment. The therapeutic relationship in CBT is described as being one of *collaborative empiricism*, where the therapist assumes the role of a coach or teacher in addition to providing the more traditional nonspecific elements of empathy, understanding, and support. Through this model of interaction the therapist and patient develop step-wise goals to reduce symptoms, improve management of pressing day-to-day problems, and increase morale. Collaboration is explicitly fostered via the use of summarization and feedback to ensure that the patient thoroughly understands the material being covered. CBT also draws heavily on the principles and methods of behavior therapy, including activity scheduling, graded task assignments, guided practice, and individualized homework assignments. Explicit, step-wise strategies are used to improve recognition of problem areas and effect changes in thoughts, behaviors, and feelings. As with other types of psychotherapy, the establishment of a strong therapeutic relationship based upon warmth, empathy, and genuineness is crucial to obtaining positive outcomes. A strong therapeutic alliance enhances learning and the mastery of targeted therapeutic tasks. Compared with the process of more traditional dynamic therapies, CBT requires greater therapist activity.

Furthermore, CBT differs from dynamic or experiential therapies in that affect is specifically used to identify a cognitive process by which depressed patients learn to solve problems and gain greater control over dysphoric and anhedonic moods. Like IPT, typical CBT treatment of acute depression involves 12–14 therapy sessions over a 3- to 4-month period. Longer-term CBT therapy can be useful for prevention of relapse of acute depressive episodes, and to revise core beliefs and dysfunctional behavioral patterns in individuals with longstanding personality or characterologic disorders.

## Combination psychotherapy and psychopharmacotherapy for depression

The goal of both psychotherapy and pharmacological treatment is to eliminate all manifestations of disorder, but individuals frequently do not achieve adequate clinical response, and relapse and recurrence are common [4]. Often referred to as "combined" or "combination" treatment, psychiatric treatment utilizing both psychotherapy and pharmacology is frequently used in practice to treat depression [1,5,6]. There are several different definitions of "combined" treatment; for example, the combination of treatment can be offered simultaneously or additively. Additive treatment can be in one of two sequential orders: psychotherapy (either individual or group) first augmented by medication or pharmacological treatment supplemented by therapy. Combined treatment can be "split" and provided by multiple providers, or integrated, with the psychiatrist providing both treatments.

Lacking a strong empirical basis, much of the existing literature discussing the pros and cons of combined treatment is based on clinical opinion and theoretical speculation. The prevailing arguments for and against combining therapy and medication are highlighted in Figure 6.1. There are a growing number of clinical trials showing combined treatment to be superior to either type of intervention used alone for depression [5,7]. Nevertheless, expert consensus panels have recommended combination treatment for the treatment of depression, especially

| Pros and cons of combined psychotherapy and pharmacology | | | |
|---|---|---|---|
| Adding pharmacology | | Adding psychotherapy | |
| Pros | Cons | Pros | Cons |
| Provides symptom relief and helps patients engage better in therapy (e.g., improve concentration, hyperarousal, or decrease fatigue). Stabilizes ego functions to enable better psychotherapy participation<br><br>May increase positive expectancy of therapy (placebo effect)<br><br>Decreases distorted or irrational thinking that interferes with therapy progress | Prematurely decreases target symptoms and decreases motivation for therapy or to learn new ways to cope without medication<br><br>May imply to patients that they cannot handle their disease<br><br>Elicits negative transference reactions or undercuts psychological defenses<br><br>Medications can interfere with learning and memory or cause "state-dependent" learning in therapy<br><br>Increases risk of relapse if discontinued, which may negatively impact on prevention efforts of therapy | Helps with medication management and improves compliance<br><br>May increase positive expectancy of medication (placebo effect)<br><br>Decreases risk of relapse of psychiatric disorder<br><br>Improves social and occupational functioning<br><br>Lessens impact of psychosocial stressors and allows patient to gain self-understanding of more adaptive coping strategies | May lead therapist to ignore biological factors and place too much responsibility on the patient<br><br>Therapy could place undue stress on patients with biologically driven illness states |

Figure 6.1 Pros and cons of combined psychotherapy and pharmacology. Adapted from [6].

when the illness presentation or course is complicated [8,9]. Some circumstances in which combination treatment may be helpful include the following:

- when either treatment alone, optimally given, is only partially effective
- if the clinical circumstances suggest two discrete targets of therapy (e.g., symptom reduction addressed by medication and social/occupational problems addressed by psychotherapy)
- if the prior course of illness is chronic; for relapse prevention in patients achieving only a partial response to pharmacotherapy in the acute phase
- to aid in improving medication adherence and treatment compliance.

The intriguing findings of Mayberg and colleagues demonstrating the brain regions associated with antidepressant and CBT activity provides an explanatory model for combined treatment. Mayberg identified the prefrontal cortex as being a target of pharmacotherapy, with the highest concentration of serotonin in the brain [10]. Goldapple and co-workers analyzed patients treated with an SSRI (paroxetine) and CBT, and demonstrated that CBT is associated with characteristic metabolic changes in the frontal cortex, cingulate, and hippocampus rather than the characteristic changes in the prefrontal cortex, hippocampus, and cingulate regions that result from treatment with SSRIs [11]. Mayberg and colleagues interpret these findings as indicating that CBT and medications have different primary anatomical targets of action, with cortical "top-down" effects characterizing psychotherapy effect and subcortical "bottom-up" effects accounting for the effect of medication [10]. These imaging data lend support to a theoretical position suggesting that combination treatment of depression may be synergistic in its benefits because the different modalities affect different brain regions.

There are clinician and patient factors that influence the use of combination treatments. Clinicians have theoretical biases that can influence the therapeutic process during combination treatment, some oriented by preference and training to practice a specific form of psychotherapy, such as psychoanalysis, CBT, or IPT. These clinicians may view psychotherapy as the primary treatment modality with pharmacological agents being used adjunctively. For psychoanalysts, obstacles to combination treatment may include the following:

- maintaining their theoretical orientation while assessing the benefit from adjunctive medication
- a relative inexperience with medication treatments
- a lack of role models for combined treatment.

From a CBT perspective, the focus of combined treatment is the synergistic use of each modality to maximize the effect of the other modality. For a psychopharmacologically oriented psychiatrist, psychotherapy may be seen as a modality to primarily augment the use of medication. Although there may be disagreement about which approach is the most clinically efficacious, most psychiatrists agree that, optimally, combining modalities should be complementary and improve overall patient care. Another critical factor to consider in evaluating whether combination treatment should be used is patient expectation and acceptance of two treatments. It is important to explore patients' understanding of treatment options, their objections to different components, and depression treatments available to them. Providing psychoeducation about combination treatment may also minimize medication noncompliance and improve treatment adherence. Thus, the examination of interpersonal, emotional, and cognitive obstacles to treatment may promote more positive pharmacological outcomes. Fostering the patient's readiness to change and strengthening the doctor–patient alliance are important factors mediating the efficacy of medication treatment. In conclusion, the delivery of combined treatment is often complicated by multiple providers, and the expectancies of patients and the providers, each bringing their own life experiences, expectations, fears, funds of knowledge, and theoretical biases to the treatment setting.

## Physical treatments

In addition to pharmacological and psychological treatments of depression, there are a number of physical treatments (e.g., electroconvulsive therapy [ECT], phototherapy, and acupuncture) with evidence for their use. There are also several experimental stimulation treatments for depression that are currently under study, including vagus nerve stimulation (VNS), transcranial magnetic stimulation (TMS), and deep brain stimulation (DBS).

### Electroconvulsive therapy

ECT has been proven to be a safe and effective treatment for depression, and has been used successfully for more than 70 years [13]. Several recent, large-scale, multisite, collaborative studies have confirmed the efficacy of ECT for depression. In the Consortium for Research in ECT (CORE) study, 217 individuals with major depression received a course of ECT; the investigators reported a remission rate of 75% at completion and 65% at 4 weeks [14]. Similarly, another multisite collaborative study of 290 depressed individuals receiving ECT reported a remission rate of 55%. In another study, the CORE investigators examined whether receiving an additional 10 treatments of ECT or continuation pharmacotherapy improved rates of relapse over 6 months of follow-up. They found no difference between the treatments, with a third relapsing and less than half remaining well, and concluded that both treatments had limited efficacy [15]. The UK ECT Review Group (2003) performed a systematic review and meta-analysis of short-term efficacy from randomized controlled ECT trials. They report that real ECT was significantly more effective than simulated (sham) ECT (6 trials, 256 patients, standardized effect size [SES] −0.91, 95% CI −1.27 to −0.54), treatment with ECT was significantly more effective than pharmacotherapy (18 trials, 1144 participants, SES −0.80, 95% CI −1.29 to −0.29), and bilateral electrode placement was more effective

**Psychological treatment for mild, moderate, or severe depression**

Improving symptoms
*Likely to be beneficial:*
- CT (mild-to-moderate depression)
- ITP (mild-to-moderate depression)
- Combining antidepressants and psychological treatment (mild-to-moderate and severe depression)

*Unknown effectiveness:*
- Befriending (mild-to-moderate depression)
- Problem-solving therapy (mild-to-moderate depression)
- Nondirective counselling (mild-to-moderate depression)

Reducing relapse rate
*Unknown effectiveness:*
- CT (weak evidence for reduced relapse rates 1–2 years after mild-to-moderate depression)
- Relapse prevention program (no significant difference in response rates)

Figure 6.2 Psychological treatment for mild, moderate, or severe depression. CT, cognitive therapy; IPT, interpersonal therapy. Adapted from [12].

than unipolar (22 trials, 1408 participants, SES −0.32, 95% CI −0.46 to −0.19) [16]. Another meta-analytic review of randomized controlled ECT trials compared ECT with simulated ECT, placebo, or antidepressants. They found a significant superiority of ECT in all comparisons: ECT versus simulated ECT, ECT versus placebo, ECT versus antidepressants in general, ECT versus TCAs, and ECT versus MAOIs. In addition, they compared nonrandomized controlled ECT trials and found a significant statistical difference in favor of ECT versus antidepressants. They suggest that ECT is a valid therapeutic tool for treatment of depression, including severe and resistant forms [17].

The American Psychiatric Association (APA) Task Force on ECT [18] provides a good review of current clinical standards for the treatment, training, and privileging of ECT treatment [19]. The primary indications for treatment are a lack of response or intolerance to antidepressants, a previous good response to ECT, the need for a rapid treatment response because of psychosis or risk of suicide, or the presence of extremely severe or chronic depression. Clinicians must review with the patient and/or family members appropriate alternative treatments, and evaluate the risks and benefits of ECT treatment for the individual. Factors associated with reduced ECT efficacy include prolonged duration of the current depressive episode, lack of response to medication, and the presence of a comorbid personality disorder [13]. There are no absolute contraindications, although those with unstable cardiac disease (e.g., ischemia or arrhythmia), cerebrovascular disease (e.g., recent cerebral hemorrhage or stroke), or increased intracranial pressure are at increased risk for complications [20].

## Phototherapy

Phototherapy – the use of light treatment – was developed to treat, and has become the first-line treatment for, individuals with seasonal affective disorder (SAD) [21]. Meta-analysis has confirmed the efficacy of light therapy in the treatment of seasonal and nonseasonal depression with effect sizes equivalent to that of most antidepressant pharmaceutical trials [22], although caution is warranted as the quality of studies included is poor. In addition, it has shown efficacy for the treatment of premenstrual [23] and antepartum depression [24]. Three of four SAD sufferers are women and the usual age of onset is between 18 and 30 years [25]. As is characteristic for the disorder, winter seasonal depression spontaneously remits in the spring and summer (less frequently, some individuals have a depressive pattern characterized by summer depression and spontaneous winter remission). The most common form of phototherapy is white light treatment of 2500–10,000 lux (equaling the light exposure of a bright sunny day). Phototherapy has been recommended as a first-line treatment for SAD (APA, 2000). There is also evidence that phototherapy may accelerate remission in nonseasonal depression together with medication [23].

In 1980, Lewy and colleagues were the first to recognize that melatonin could be suppressed with bright light. Melatonin is believed to regulate circadian rhythmicity and bright light appears to be responsible for melatonin suppression, the key regulatory mechanism for maintaining normal biological rhythms. Thus, phototherapy appears to aid maintenance of normal biological rhythmicity by compensating for circadian phase advances in the sleep cycle (through late afternoon exposure) and for phase delays (through early morning exposure) [26].

In addition, some investigators propose that phototherapy also affects neurotransmitter function and that this may also contribute to its antidepressant activity in vulnerable individuals [27].

## Other physical treatments

Similar to ECT, these treatments use devices to introduce an electrical current that theoretically alters neuronal circuits. Positive outcomes with surgical lesion procedures since the 1940s to interrupt brain circuits (such as anterior cingulotomy and subcaudate tractotomy) suggest a role for stimulation treatments that are less invasive for severe and treatment-resistant MDDs. The stimulation treatments utilize focused excitation of brain regions to, theoretically, produce a desired behavioral alteration. Models of limbic–cortical dysfunction in MDD have been proposed that characterize the depression phenotype at the neural systems level [28] and provide a theoretical basis for neuromodulation treatments. Studies are now in progress on a number of different therapeutic neuromodulation treatments.

## Vagus nerve stimulation

In 2005, VNS was approved by the FDA for individuals with treatment-resistant depression [29]. It had previously been approved for use as an adjunctive therapy for epilepsy. VNS requires a surgically implanted, battery-powered pulse generator and electrical lead wound around the left vagus nerve. This provides intermittent stimulation, typically 30 seconds on and 5 minutes off. The most common adverse effects are voice alteration during stimulation and hoarseness, dyspnea, and cough. Hypomania may be a treatment-induced adverse effect and there is a risk of surgical infection. The device is programmed using an external programming system to alter the generator output. VNS stimulation did not demonstrate acute phase efficacy in one small open-label study (18 of 59 responded positively) [30], but has shown promising results to suggest benefit to patients with low-to-moderate degrees of treatment resistance and over longer-term treatment [31]. A 12-month, nonrandomized study of similar type treatment-resistant patients compared VNS treatment plus treatment-as-usual to treatment-as-usual alone and found significantly greater symptomatic benefit in the VNS group [32]. Nahas et al. reported that, after 2 years of VNS treatment, the response rate was 42% and remission rate 22%, and that 81% were still actively using the device (implying that those who did not reach response criteria still perceived a subjective benefit from the device)[33]. Currently, a large multisite study is under way to assess VNS efficacy at several different generator settings.

## Transcranial magnetic stimulation

TMS has been used to treat patients who have not benefited sufficiently from pharmacotherapy and psychotherapy. TMS is applied without sedation, externally delivering the stimulation to the brain through the cranium. Several small (usually single-site), sham-controlled trials of TMS and meta-analysis of their results support its efficacy for the treatment of MDD [34]. Recently, a double-blind, multisite study trial of over 300 medication-free patients with major depression were randomized to active or sham TMS. Sessions were conducted five times a week for 4–6 weeks. Active TMS was significantly superior to sham TMS, with remission rates approximately twofold higher for active TMS, and active TMS was well tolerated with a low dropout rate for adverse events (generally mild and limited to transient scalp discomfort or pain). The investigators report a small effect size with an NNT of 11 – roughly comparable to NNT values reported for antidepressant medications [35]. To date, the existing literature suggests a potential role for TMS for depressed individuals with treatment-resistant depression, but the optimum treatment parameters remain to be established. A commercial TMS device was FDA approved for treatment of depression in the USA in October 2008, becoming the second stimulation treatment thus far approved for depression treatment in the USA.

### Deep brain stimulation

DBS also has FDA approval for the treatment of epilepsy and is being studied for the treatment of depression [36]. In DBS, electrodes are surgically implanted in the subgenual cingulate area, also known as Brodmann area 25. This area of the anterior cingulate cortex has been shown to be metabolically overactive in patients with depression or in healthy individuals who are induced to feel sad. This area is thought to be involved in cortisol regulation, stress response, sleep modulation, emotional regulation of the limbic system, motivation, and drive. Mayberg and colleagues found that chronic stimulation of white matter tracts adjacent to the subgenual cingulate gyrus was associated with a striking and sustained remission of depression in four of six patients participating in an open-label trial [37]. Antidepressant effects were associated with a marked reduction in local cerebral blood flow as well as changes in downstream limbic and cortical sites, measured using positron emission tomography. The authors suggest that disruption of focal pathological activity in limbic–cortical circuits, using electrical stimulation of the subgenual cingulate white matter, can effectively reverse symptoms in otherwise treatment-resistant depression. Such preliminary findings are promising and further, confirmatory, studies are currently under way. Adverse effects of DBS include surgical risks, such as infection, hemorrhage, and seizure, and a risk of infection from the subcutaneously planted battery and wires. Mood-related risks include the induction of hypomania. Stimulation-associated adverse effects include sensorimotor changes, insomnia, autonomic changes (e.g., transient increases in heart rate and blood pressure), and memory flashbacks.

## Lifestyle and complementary therapies

Many individuals with mild-to-moderately severe depressive episodes seek lifestyle and complementary therapies, such as exercise, hypericum extracts (St John's wort), and omega-3-fatty acids (O-3-FA).

## Exercise

There have been a few RCTs addressing the use of exercise to treat depression. Dunn and colleagues performed a randomized, placebo-controlled, 12-week study in adults (age 20–45 years) with MDDs to determine if higher total energy expenditure and frequency of exercise improved depressive symptoms and, if so, whether there is an exercise dose–response relationship [38]. They reported that increasing energy expenditure (by >17.5 kcal/kg per week) significantly reduced depressive symptoms, but there was no main effect of exercise frequency. They concluded that aerobic exercise at a dose consistent with public health recommendations is an effective treatment for MDDs of mild-to-moderate severity [38]. Blumenthal and colleagues performed a prospective RCT involving 202 adults with major depression who were treated with group-supervised exercise, home-based exercise, antidepressant (sertraline 50–200 mg daily), or placebo. After 4 months, patients who received active treatments tended ($p=0.057$) to have higher remission rates than those on placebo. These authors conclude that the efficacy of exercise seems to be generally comparable to antidepressant treatment [39]. In an earlier report, Babyak et al. followed individuals who completed the above study and found that fewer in the exercise group relapsed over the next 6 months [40].

Exercise has also been examined as an augmentation treatment for depression. Trivedi and colleagues examined the use of exercise to augment SSRI treatment in 17 MDD patients with incomplete remission of depressive symptoms [41]. Patients underwent a 12-week individualized exercise program while continuing their antidepressant (unchanged in type or dose). Intent-to-treat analyses yielded significant decreases in depressive symptoms. This study provides preliminary evidence for exercise as an effective augmentation treatment for antidepressants. These investigators suggest that exercise is a lower-cost augmentation strategy with numerous health benefits, and it may further reduce depressive symptoms in those who partially respond to antidepressants [41].

Lawlor and Hopter performed a systematic review and meta-regression analysis of RCTs of exercise as an intervention in the management of depression [42]. Hampered by poor-quality evidence they, nevertheless, found that the difference in effect sizes between exercise and CBT (four studies) was not significant. Similarly, in the study comparing exercise and antidepressant, or both, there was no significant difference in outcomes between treatments. As with the case for acupuncture treatment for depression, the preliminary evidence argues for additional studies to validate these preliminary findings [42].

## St John's wort

St John's wort (*Hypericum perforatum*) is the herbal therapy most commonly available worldwide for the treatment of depression. Its main active principle has not yet been identified and preparations of this compound are often unstandardized. It can interact with antidepressants acting on the 5HT system, such as SSRIs. Adverse effects are generally mild.

A number of clinical trials suggest that St John's wort may enhance 5HT function and be effective in the treatment of mild-to-moderate depression. Linde and colleagues performed a systematic review and meta-analysis to investigate if extracts of *H. perforatum* are more effective and more tolerable than placebo and antidepressants in the treatment of depression [43]. They reviewed 23 randomized trials (total of 1757 outpatients) in patients with mild or moderately severe depressive disorders. They report that *Hypericum* extracts were significantly superior to placebo and as effective as standard antidepressants, and concluded that there is evidence for *Hypericum* extracts being more effective than placebo for treatment of mildly to moderately severe depression [43]. A more recent, double-blind RCT of *Hypericum* extract compared with fluoxetine and placebo in 135 patients with major depression found that *Hypericum* was significantly more effective than fluoxetine and tended toward superiority over placebo. However, this study was compromised by the limitation of the dosage of fluoxetine to 20 mg/day, the low end of its recommended sp -prescribing range (20–60 mg/day) [44].

A review of other recent trials continues to provide inconclusive evidence about *Hypericum*'s efficacy for depression. Shelton et al. studied 200 outpatients with major depression and reported *Hypericum* not to be effective compared with placebo [45]. This group examined the 95 patients who did not respond and found them not to be highly treatment resistant, further arguing against its efficacy versus antidepressants [46]. The Hypericum Depression Study Group trial [47] performed a multisite study with 340 depressed individuals comparing *Hypericum* with placebo and sertraline; they report that this study failed to support its use. On the other hand, reports by Kasper et al. [48] and Lecrubier et al. [49] found it to be safe and more effective than placebo.

## Omega-3-fatty acids

The family of O-3-FAs includes eicosapentaenoic acid (EPA) and docosahexaenoic acid (DHA). Greater dietary intakes of O-3-FAs may be beneficial for depressed mood and have generated interest in their use as an antidepressant treatment. However, at present, it is unclear whether they have a potential role [50]; for example, one randomized, double-blind, clinical trial of DHA in

36 individuals with major depression failed to find a significant effect of DHA monotherapy [50]. Another randomized trial examined the efficacy of EPA in treating depression in those with bipolar depression. In a 12-week, double-blind study, participants were randomly assigned to adjunctive treatment with placebo or two doses of EPA. They reported significant improvement with EPA compared with placebo and both doses were well tolerated [4].

Sontrop and Campbell evaluated the evidence for the efficacy of O-3-FAs in patients with unipolar and postpartum depression [51]. They note that studies in this area are confounded by a lack of power or incomplete control. In four of seven double-blind RCTs reviewed by these authors, depression was significantly improved with O-3-FA. However, although clinical significance was demonstrated, preservation of blinding may have been a major limitation, making it unclear whether O-3-FA supplementation is effective independently of antidepressant treatment for depressed patients in general, or only for those with abnormally low concentrations of these O-3-FAs [51].

Lin and colleagues performed a systematic review and meta-analysis of clinical trials in the English literature of O-3-FA efficacy. A total of 10 double-blind, placebo-controlled studies in patients with mood disorders receiving O-3-FAs for 4 weeks or longer were included. They found a significant antidepressant effect for O-3-FAs in unipolar and bipolar depression. However, significant heterogeneity among these studies and publication bias were noted, with the conclusion that it is still premature to validate this finding [52]. Similarly, Appleton et al. reviewed 18 RCTs and included 12 in a meta-analysis. They concluded that the evidence examining the effects of O-3-FAs on depressed mood is limited, and difficult to summarize and evaluate because of considerable heterogeneity [53]. Furthermore, the available evidence provides little support for the use of O-3-FAs to improve depressed mood, and suggests that larger trials with adequate power to detect clinically important benefits are required to help clarify this issue.

## Acupuncture

Despite its being practiced for thousands of years, there is little evidence supporting the use of acupuncture in the English-speaking medical literature, and only uncontrolled trials for acupuncture for treatments of illnesses that prominently include depression in Chinese and Russian reports [54]. Allen and colleagues examined the effectiveness of acupuncture for depression versus acupuncture treatment of nonspecific symptoms and a waiting-list condition in a small sample of 38 women with major depression. After 8 weeks of treatment, there was a statistically significant difference ($p<0.05$) between the specific versus nonspecific acupuncture treatment, but only a marginal difference ($p > 0.12$) between the specific treatment and the waiting-list control [55]. However, effect size calculations show that the specific treatment had a large effect size ($d = 1.16$, where $d$ is Cohen's $d$) compared with nonspecific treatment, which, in turn, had a moderate-to-large effect size compared with waiting list ($d = 0.61$) suggesting an effect comparable to standard treatments such as psychotherapy and pharmacotherapy [55].

Smith and Hay performed a Cochrane Database Systematic Review of acupuncture studies for depression, including all published and unpublished RCTs comparing acupuncture with sham acupuncture, no treatment, pharmacological treatment, other structured psychotherapies (CBT, psychotherapy, or counseling), or standard care [56]. The participants included men and women with depression (defined by clinical state description, or diagnosed by DSM-IV or ICD criteria). The primary outcomes were reduction in depression severity measured by self or clinician rating scales and rates of remission versus nonremission. Meta-analysis was performed using seven trials comprising 517 participants. Five trials (409 participants) included a comparison between acupuncture and medication. Two other trials compared acupuncture with a waiting-list control or sham acupuncture. Participants generally had mild-to-moderate depression. There was no evidence that medication was better than acupuncture in reducing the severity of depression (weighted mean difference 0.53, 95% CI –1.42 to +2.47), or in improving depression, defined as remission versus no remission (RR 1.2, 95% CI 0.94–1.51). The authors conclude that there is insufficient evidence to determine the efficacy of acupuncture compared with medication, waiting-list control, or sham acupuncture [56].

In summary, the limitations of the current acupuncture studies (diagnostic imprecision, variation in the treatment provision, and small sample size) compromise our ability to determine its true effectiveness compared with other depression treatments, and further study is needed.

## References

1 Friedman ES, Thase ME. Depression-focused psychotherapies. In: Treatment of Psychiatric Disorders, Vol 2, 4th edition. Edited by GO Gabbard. Washington, DC: American Psychiatric Press, Inc, 2007; 409–431.
2 Beck AT, Rush AJ, Shaw BF, et al. Cognitive Therapy of Depression. New York: Guilford, 1979.
3 Klerman GL, Weissman MM, Rounsaville BJ, et al. Interpersonal Psychotherapy of Depression. New York: Basic Books, 1984.
4 Frangou S, Lewis M, McCrone P. Efficacy of ethyl-eicosapentaenoic acid in bipolar depression: randomised double-blind placebo-controlled study. Br J Psychiatry 2006; 188:46–50.
5 Friedman ES, Wright JH, Jarrett RB, et al. Combining cognitive therapy and medication for mood disorders. Psychiatr Ann 2006; 36:320–328.
6 Szigethy EM, Friedman ES. Combined psychotherapy and pharmacotherapy. In: Comprehensive Textbook of Psychiatry IX. Edited by HI Kaplan & BJ Zaddock. Baltimore, MD: Williams & Wilkins, 2009: in press.
7 Pampelloma S, Bollini P, Tibaldi G, et al. Combined pharmacotherapy and psychological treatment for depression: a systematic review. Arch Gen Psychiatry 2004; 61:714–719.
8 AHCPR Depression Guideline Panel. Depression in Primary Care, Vol 1. Detection and diagnosis. Clinical practice guideline 5. Rockville, MD: US Department of Health and Human Services, Public Health Service, Agency for Health Care Policy and Research, 1993.
9 American Psychiatric Association. Practice guideline for the treatment of patients with major depressive disorder (revision). Am J Psychiatry 2000; 157(Suppl 4):1–45.
10 Mayberg HS. Modulating dysfunctional limbic–cortical circuits in depression: towards development of brain-based algorithms for diagnosis and optimised treatment. Br Med Bull 2003; 65:193–207.
11 Goldapple K, Segal Z, Garson C, et al. Modulation of cortical–limbic pathways in major depression: treatment-specific effects of cognitive behavior therapy. Arch Gen Psychiatry 2004; 61:34–41.
12 Butler R, Hatcher S, Price J, et al. Depression in adults: psychological treatments and care pathways. BMJ Clin Evidence 2007; 1016:1–18.
13 Prudic J, Olfson M, Marcus SC, et al. Effectiveness of electroconvulsive therapy in community settings. Biol Psychiatry 2004; 55:301–312.
14 Husain MM, Rush AJ, Fink M, et al. Speed of response and remission in major depressive disorder with acute electroconvulsive therapy (ECT): a Consortium for Research in ECT (CORE) report. J Clin Psychiatry 2004; 65:485–491.
15 Kellner CH, Knapp RG, Petrides G, et al. Continuation electroconvulsive therapy vs pharmacotherapy for relapse prevention in major depression: a multisite study from the consortium for research in electroconvulsive therapy (CORE). Arch Gen Psychiatry 2006; 63:1337–1344.
16 UK ECT Review Group. Efficacy and safety of electroconvulsive therapy in depressive disorders: a systematic review and meta-analysis. Lancet 2003; 361:799–808.
17 Pagnin D, de Queiroz V, Pini S. Efficacy of ECT in depression: a meta-analytic review. J ECT 2004; 20:13–20.
18 Weiner RD. Practice of Electroconvulsive Therapy: Recommendations for Treatment, Training, and Privileging, 2nd edition. Task Force Report of the American Psychiatric Association. Washington, DC: American Psychiatric Publishing, Inc, 2001.
19 Scott AIF. The ECT Handbook: The Third Report of the Royal College of Psychiatrists' Special Committee on ECT (Council Report CR128), 2nd edition. London, UK; Royal College of Psychiatry 2005.
20 Lisenby SH. Electroconvulsive therapy for depression. N Eng J Med 2007; 357:1939–1945.

21 Partonen T, Magnusson A (eds). Seasonal Affective Disorder. Practice and Research. Oxford, UK: Oxford University Press, 2001.
22 Golden RN, Gaynes BN, Ekstrom RD, et al. The efficacy of light therapy in the treatment of mood disorders: a review and meta-analysis of the evidence. Am J Psychiatry 2005; 162:656–662.
23 Lam RW. Seasonal Affective Disorder and Beyond. Light Treatment for SAD and nonSAD conditions. Washington, DC: American Psychiatric Press, 1998.
24 Epperson CN, Terman M, Terman JS, et al. Randomized clinical trial of bright light therapy for antepartum depression: preliminary findings. J Clin Psychiatry 2004; 65:421–425.
25 Rosenthal NE, Blehar MC. Seasonal Affective Disorders and Phototherapy. New York: Guilford, 1989.
26 Lewy AJ, Wehr TA, Goodwin DA, et al. Light suppresses melatonin secretion in humans. Science 1980; 210:1267–1269.
27 Lam RW, Tam EM, Yatham LN, et al. Seasonal depression: the dual vulnerability hypothesis revisited. J Affect Disord 2001; 63:123–132.
28 Seminowicz DA, Mayberg HS, McIntosh AR, et al. Limbic–frontal circuitry in major depression: a path modeling meta-analysis. Neuroimage 2004; 22:409–418.
29 Shuchman M. Approving the vagus-nerve stimulator for depression. N Engl J Med 2007; 356:1604–1607.
30 Rush AJ, Marangell LB, Sackeim HA, et al. Vagus nerve stimulation for treatment-resistant depression: a randomized, controlled acute phase trial. Biol Psychiatry 2005; 58:347–354.
31 Sackeim HA, Rush AJ, George MS, et al. Vagus nerve stimulation (VNS) for treatment resistant depression: efficacy, side effects and predictors of outcome. Neuropsychopharmacology 2001; 25:713–728.
32 George MS, Rush AJ, Marengell LA, et al. One-year comparison of vagus nerve stimulation with treatment as usual for treatment-resistant depression. Biol Psychiatry 2005; 58:364–373.
33 Nahas Z, Marangell LB, Husain MM, et al. Two-year outcome of vagus-nerve stimulation (VNS) for treatment of major depressive episodes. J Clin Psychiatry 2005; 66:1097–1104.
34 Janicak PG, O'Reardon JP, Sampson SM, et al. Transcranial magnetic stimulation in the treatment of major depressive disorder: a comprehensive summary of safety experience from acute exposure, extended exposure, and during reintroduction treatment. J Clin Psychiatry 2008; 69:222–232.
35 Thase ME, Haight BR, Richard N, et al. Remission rates following antidepressant therapy with bupropion or selective serotonin reuptake inhibitors: a meta-analysis of original data from 7 randomized controlled trials. J Clin Psychiatry 2005; 66:974–81.
36 Anderson I, Ferrier I, Baldwin R, et al. Evidence-based guidelines for treating depressive disorders with antidepressants: a revision of the 2000 British Association for Psychopharmacology guidelines. J Psychopharmacol 2008; 22:343–396.
37 Mayberg HS, Lozano AM, Voon V, et al. Deep brain stimulation for treatment-resistant depression. Neuron 2005; 45:651–60.
38 Dunn AL, Trivedi MH, Kampert JB, et al. Exercise treatment for depression: efficacy and dose response. Am J Prev Med 2005; 28:140–141.
39 Blumenthal JA, Sherwood A, Rogers SD, et al. Understanding prognostic benefits of exercise and antidepressant therapy for persons with depression and heart disease: the UPBEAT study – rationale, design, and methodological issues. Clin Trials 2007; 4:548–559.
40 Babyak M, Blumenthal JA, Herman S, et al. Exercise treatment for major depression: maintenance of therapeutic benefit at 10 months. Psychosom Med 2000; 62:633–638.
41 Trivedi MH, Greer TL, Grannemann BD, et al. Exercise as an augmentation strategy. Psychiatr Pract 2006; 12:205–213.
42 Lawlor DA, Hopter SW. The effectiveness of exercise as an intervention in the management of depression: systematic review and meta-regression analysis of randomised controlled trials. BMJ 2001; 322:1–8.

43 Linde K, Ramirez G, Cynthia D, et al. St John's wort for depression – an overview and meta-analysis of randomised clinical trials. BMJ 1996; 313:253–258.
44 Fava M, Alpert J, Nierenberg AA, et al. A double-blind, randomized trial of St John's wort, fluoxetine, and placebo in major depressive disorder. J Clin Psychopharmacol 2005; 25:441–447.
45 Shelton RC, Keller MB, Gelenberg AJ, et al. Effectiveness of St. John's Wort in major depression: a randomized controlled trial. JAMA 2001; 285:1978–1986.
46 Gelenberg AJ, Shelton RC, Crits-Christoph P, et al. The effectiveness of St. John's Wort in major depressive disorder: a naturalistic phase 2 follow-up in which nonresponders were provided alternate medication. J Clin Psychiatry 2004; 65:1114–1119.
47 Hypericum Depression Study Group. Effect of *Hypericum perforatum* (St John's wort) in major depressive disorder. JAMA 2002; 287:1807–1814.
48 Kasper S, Anghelescu IG, Szegedi A, et al. Superior efficacy of St John's wort extract WS 55 70 compared to placebo in patients with major depression: a randomized, double-blind, placebo-controlled, multi-center trial [ISRCTN77277298]. BMC Med 2006; 4:14.
49 Lecrubier Y, Clerc G, Didi R, et al. Efficacy of St John's wort extract WS 5570 in major depression: a double-blind, placebo-controlled trial. Am J Psychiatry 2002; 159:1361–1366.
50 Marangell LB, Martinez JM, Zboyan HA, et al. A double-blind, placebo-controlled study of the omega-3 fatty acid docosahexaenoic acid in the treatment of major depression. Am J Psychiatry 2003; 160:996–998.
51 Sontrop J, Campbell MK. Omega-3 polyunsaturated fatty acids and depression: a review of the evidence and a methodological critique. Prev Med 2006; 42:4–13.
52 Lin PY, Su KP. A meta-analytic review of double-blind, placebo-controlled trials of antidepressant efficacy of omega-3 fatty acids. J Clin Psychiatry 2007; 68:1056–1061.
53 Appleton KM, Hayward RC, Gunnell D, et al. Effects of n-3 long-chain polyunsaturated fatty acids on depressed mood: systematic review of published trials. Am J Clin Nutr 2007; 84:1308–1316.
54 Allen JJB. Depression and acupuncture: a controlled clinical trial. Elements Health Centre 2000; 17:1–4.
55 Allen JJB, Schnyer RN, Hitt SK. The efficacy of acupuncture in the treatment of major depression in women. Psychol Sci 1998; 9:397–401.
56 Smith CA, Hay PP. Acupuncture for depression. Cochrane Database System Rev 2005; (2): CD004046.

# Chapter 7

## Management of treatment nonresponse

Ian M Anderson

Inadequate treatment response is unfortunately a common problem. Approximately 50–70% of patients gain significant benefit from treatment but, of these, not all will have symptomatic remission [1]. An approximate rule of thirds applies, with a third achieving remission, a third being significantly better but not symptom free with partial remission, and a third remaining depressed. These proportions depend on the duration of follow-up and the nature of the population being studied. Consideration of next-step treatments is therefore extremely important and a pessimist might say that the next step should be planned at the time of the first step. It is certainly important to plan treatment in the knowledge that further steps might be needed.

### Assessment and principles of management

#### Assessment

If a patient has not improved sufficiently it is important to assess the stage of treatment and timing (see Figure 4.11). An important decision is whether to continue for longer with the present treatment or make a change, which depends on the trajectory of the depressive episode, likelihood of remaining symptomatic, and functional impairment and treatment history for that patient. Although the goal of remission should always be in mind, the management is different for someone in a first episode than for someone with highly recurrent depression, a long treatment history, and incomplete interepisode recovery. In the latter case, longer periods of treatment before making changes are appropriate.

In assessing inadequate response (Figure 7.1) the aims are to re-evaluate the diagnosis and treatment goals, identify factors that may be impairing response to treatment, and identify further treatment options.

E. Friedman and I.M. Anderson, *Managing Depression in Clinical Practice*
DOI 10.1007/978-1-84996-465-4_7, © Springer-Verlag London Limited 2010

| The assessment of inadequate response to treatment | |
|---|---|
| Patient and illness factors | Check diagnosis and comorbidity<br>Exclude comorbid substance misuse<br>Check for maintaining factors:<br>- life events<br>- social support<br>- problems<br>- avoidance behavior<br>Check for physical illness<br>Review current level of depression in context of depression history and realistic treatment goals (involving patient's perspective) |
| Treatment factors | Adherence to treatment<br>Treatment adequacy (dose of antidepressant, frequency of therapy)<br>Past treatment efficacy and tolerability<br>Treatment options not tried |

Figure 7.1 The assessment of inadequate response to treatment

## Principles of management

It is possible to get caught up in making too frequent changes in treatment because of the desire by both the clinician and the patient for the latter to get better as soon as possible. At the other extreme, patients not responding to treatment can be left for too long on the same treatment and denied potentially beneficial alternatives. There must be a happy medium so that it can be established whether or not a treatment produces benefit before moving on to further planned treatment trials. This may require up to about 12 weeks per treatment trial.

The treatment strategies and suggested guidance for their use are outlined in Figure 7.2 and discussed below.

| Treatment strategies for inadequate response | |
|---|---|
| Strategy | When to consider |
| Continue current treatment | Possible trajectory of improvement still present, good tolerability, and resistant to previous treatments |
| Increase dose | Scope for dose increase, good tolerability, and possible slight improvement |
| Switch treatment | No improvement in spite of adequate treatment, poor tolerability |
| Add second treatment | Some improvement, good tolerability if second drug to be added |

Figure 7.2 Treatment strategies for inadequate response. Adapted from [2].

Patient choice is important because many will have preferred options at this stage. They may be reluctant to continue the current treatment or increase dose because of side effects; alternatively they may be reluctant to stop because of a wish not to lose the gains made. On current evidence we have little to guide the choice of next-step treatment and there are no convincing differences in efficacy between strategies, or between most choices within a strategy. Most evidence that we have is for antidepressants and next-step treatment with psychological treatments has been little studied.

## Definitions: treatment nonresponse and treatment-resistant depression

Nonresponse can be technically defined as less than 50% improvement in the initial rating scale score (see Chapter 4). This is of limited clinical use and it is better to consider the severity of continuing symptoms and functional impairment in consultation with the patient when determining what is better termed "inadequate response or improvement."

Treatment-resistant depression (TRD) has become an accepted term and is commonly taken to mean failure to respond to two or more treatments given at an adequate dose for an adequate length of time. Exact definitions vary but the common stages are given in Figure 7.3. However, the term "TRD" is less useful than it appears at first sight: as usually applied, it does not include partial remission; it is difficult to incorporate psychological treatments into the definition; defining what counts as an adequate treatment can be difficult; and there is no natural cut-off between two or fewer treatments and three or more treatments. There is also the problem of labeling patients as being treatment-resistant in an arbitrary way. What is true is that progressively fewer people respond to subsequent treatments after previous inadequate treatment response. This has been shown most clearly in STAR*D, the largest sequencing study to date [3,4].

### Classification of treatment nonresponse/resistance

Different detailed schemes are used but in general include four stages:

1. Inadequate treatment (i.e., not really resistance to treatment)
2. Nonresponse to an adequate trial of a single agent
3. Degrees of TRD (nonresponse to adequate trials of two or more agents from different classes, augmentation, ECT)
4. Chronic refractory depression (nonresponse to multiple treatments, including augmentation and ECT)

Figure 7.3 Classification of treatment nonresponse/resistance. ECT, electroconvulsive therapy; TRD, treatment-resistant depression. Adapted from [5].

## Medication strategies

### Dose increase

Controlled studies have found no evidence that increasing the dose of SSRIs is more helpful than continuing the same dose in patients who have not responded; this is consistent with their generally flat dose–response curve [6]. There is no direct evidence for other drug classes but some do appear to have some dose–response efficacy, including the TCAs, venlafaxine, and escitalopram [6–8]. In spite of the limited evidence, increasing the dose, provided that side effects and safety allow, may be a reasonable step, especially as there is wide interindividual variability in plasma concentration of antidepressants and associated uncertainty about what is an effective dose for an individual patient. Increasing the dose may also keep a patient in treatment to allow adequate time to respond.

In patients who have failed to respond to previous treatments, high-dose antidepressants are sometimes considered. This is usually an off-label use and must be discussed with patients. Clinical experience suggests that some patients do benefit, particularly when treated with high-dose TCAs, venlafaxine, or MAOIs, but caution must be exercised and adverse events monitored (see Chapter 5).

### Switching treatment

Antidepressant switching studies show widely varying response rates (25–70%) and there is very little evidence to guide drug switching. There may be marginal benefit from switching between antidepressant classes rather than to a second drug of the same class, but this may be accounted for by studies switching from an SSRI to venlafaxine, a dual NE and serotonin reuptake inhibitor. Older studies have also suggested that switching from a reuptake inhibitor to an MAOI may be effective.

To switch safely between antidepressants there is the question of whether a wash-out period is required to avoid interactions at the cost of delay in treatment and potential deterioration in depression. Immediate switching appears reasonable with drugs of similar pharmacology, but there are also reports of safe switching between class, and indeed this may reduce discontinuation symptoms from the first drug [9]. The rule of thumb is that, if two drugs can reasonably be combined, immediate switching (between modest doses) of the two drugs appears safe and well tolerated. Potentially toxic interactions need to be considered, especially when the initial drug has long-lasting effects (e.g., fluoxetine to TCA, MAOIs to serotoninergic drugs), and it is recommended that appropriate reference books, such as the BNF or *Maudsley Prescribing Guidelines*, are consulted [10].

## Combining treatments

Adding a second agent to an antidepressant tends to be called "augmentation" when the added drug is not an antidepressant and "combination" when two antidepressants are used. The practice of combining drugs goes back to the early days of antidepressant treatment when TCAs and MAOIs were combined, a practice now viewed as without clear benefit and potentially risky.

The strongest evidence remains for lithium augmentation of monoamine reuptake inhibitors, mostly TCAs [12]. However, the studies are small and there are few recent studies, so this evidence is less secure than it once seemed. Lithium augmentation was poorly effective in the STAR*D study [3] but in other settings it does appear effective. Results with $T_3$ augmentation suggest efficacy but it has not been extensively studied and longer-term experience with continuing treatment is lacking. It was better tolerated and nonsignificantly better than lithium in the STAR*D study. In contrast, pindolol augmentation has been shown to be an ineffective strategy and RCTs with buspirone also do not support efficacy [2].

Recently studies using atypical antipsychotics as augmenting agents for SSRIs have been reported, and there is now some evidence for quetiapine, olanzapine, aripiprazole, and risperidone as effective augmenting agents, although further data are needed as well as longer-term studies. They are reasonably well tolerated but there is an increased side-effect burden [13].

The rationale behind combining antidepressants is to broaden pharmacological action in the hope that multiple actions will be of benefit. As Figure 7.4 shows, combining antidepressants appears to be relatively well tolerated and safe, provided that recognized dangers in combination are avoided (e.g., fluoxetine and paroxetine can cause high plasma TCA levels). However, evidence for efficacy is limited.

A variety of other augmentation strategies has been used. Tryptophan augmentation of MAOIs has some support and clinically it has been used as an adjunct to lithium + MAOI and lithium + TCA combinations, with the rationale that it increased serotonin availability. There is current interest in adding treatments that might be considered "complementary" to antidepressants such as EPA or folic acid, with some preliminary evidence for efficacy [2].

The disappointing efficacy of strategies for treating depression poorly responsive to antidepressants has led to a wide variety of proof-of-concept studies based on plausible pharmacological rationales. The place for these combinations is generally in research settings.

Augmentation/combination strategies are increasingly seen as a useful addition to the options for next-step treatments, but caution is warranted to ensure that they are used safely. Many combinations involve off-label use

**Efficacy and safety of drug augmentation/combination strategies**

| Combination/augmentation | Efficacy | Safety/tolerability |
|---|---|---|
| Lithium + antidepressant (mostly TCAs) | ++ | + |
| $T_3$ + antidepressants (TCAs) | + | + |
| Pindolol + antidepressants (SSRIs) | – | + |
| Buspirone + antidepressants (SSRIs) | – | + |
| Atypical antipsychotic + antidepressants (SSRIs) | + | + |
| SSRI* + mirtazapine | + | + |
| SSRI*+ bupropion (amfebutamone) | ? | + |
| SSRI*+ mianserin | (–) | + |
| SSRI*+ reboxetine | – | + |
| SSRI*+ trazodone | ? | + |
| SSRI*+ TCA | ? | + |
| Venlafaxine + mirtazapine | ? | + |
| TCA + MAOI | ? | ± |

*SSRIs that inhibit hepatic cytochrome P450 enzymes, especially fluoxetine, paroxetine, and fluvoxamine, may elevate plasma concentrations of other antidepressants.

Figure 7.4 Efficacy and safety of drug augmentation/combination strategies. ++, good evidence from meta-analysis of randomized controlled trials (RCTs); +, some evidence from RCTs for efficacy, reasonable tolerability; –, RCT evidence of lack of efficacy; (–), conflicting evidence; ?, unknown; ±, safety depends on combinations used. MAOI, monoamine oxidase inhibitors; SSRI, selective serotonin reuptake inhibitor; TCA, tricyclic antidepressant. Adapted from [2,11].

and discussion with the patient is required and informed consent obtained. Augmentation strategies are particularly useful when current treatment has produced some benefit and stopping the current antidepressant risks losing this. They are also useful when dose increase and switching strategies have failed.

## Psychological treatment strategies

There is less evidence about the use of next-step psychological treatment in patients inadequately responsive to treatment. The STAR*D study found that CBT was equally effective as antidepressants as both a switch and an augmentation strategy after inadequate response to citalopram [14]. There is some evidence that adding CBT to the treatment of patients in partial remission after being treated with antidepressants alone produces further improvement and may reduce the risk of relapse [15]. The finding that combined CBT and antidepressants may be more effective than either alone in moderate-to-severe depression adds weight to using this combination in patients inadequately responsive to either treatment alone [16,17]. At present, we do not have evidence about the place of other psychotherapies, or sequencing psychotherapies as next-step treatments.

## Physical treatment strategies

ECT is a very effective antidepressant treatment (see Chapter 6 for full discussion) and it is clear that patients who have failed to respond to a number of medication steps can derive significant benefit. One problem with using ECT in these patients is that, although acute efficacy is good, the relapse rate is high in the absence of effective continuation treatment, with up to 80% of patients relapsing over the next 6 months on placebo treatment [2]. In practice it is prudent to change the medication regimen from the one that failed before ECT and consideration should be given to augmentation with lithium.

Less established brain stimulation techniques such as repetitive TMS and VNS (see Chapter 6) may also be useful in patients who are poorly responsive to medication, although these techniques do not seem to be as effective as ECT. One study showed that VNS is unlikely to be clinically effective if there have been more than seven previous failed treatments. Another physical therapy, DBS (again discussed in Chapter 6), is currently only an experimental treatment for depression.

Ablative neurosurgery for depression has a long clinical history but there are no RCTs. Clinical experience suggests that it can be effective for some patients refractory to all other treatments. It needs to be administered in specialist centers with effective procedures for external review.

## References

1 Kennedy N, Foy K. The impact of residual symptoms on outcome of major depression. Curr Psychiatry Rep 2005;7:441–446.
2 Anderson I, Ferrier I, Baldwin R, et al. Evidence-based guidelines for treating depressive disorders with antidepressants: a revision of the 2000 British Association for Psychopharmacology guidelines. J Psychopharmacol 2008; 22:343–396.
3 Rush AJ, Trivedi MH, Wisniewski SR, et al. Acute and longer-term outcomes in depressed outpatients requiring one or several treatment steps: a STAR*D report. Am J Psychiatry 2006; 163:1905–1917.
4 Fava M. Acute and longer-term outcomes in depressed outpatients requiring one or several treatment steps: a STAR*D report. Am J Psychiatry 2006; 163:1905–1917.
5 Anderson IM. Drug treatment of depression: reflections on the evidence. Adv Psychiatr Treat 2003; 9:11–20.
6 Adli M, Baethge C, Heinz A, et al. Is dose escalation of antidepressants a rational strategy after a medium-dose treatment has failed? A systematic review. Eur Arch Psychiatry Clin Neurosci 2005; 255:387–400.
7 Rudolph RL, Fabre LF, Feighner JP, et al. A randomized, placebo-controlled, dose-response trial of venlafaxine hydrochloride in the treatment of major depression. J Clin Psychiatry 2008; 59:116–122.
8 Burke WJ, Gergel I, Bose A. Fixed-dose trial of the single isomer SSRI escitalopram in depressed outpatients. J Clin Psychiatry 2002; 63:331–336.
9 Ruhe HG, Huyser J, Swinkels JA, et al. Switching antidepressants after a first selective serotonin reuptake inhibitor in major depressive disorder: a systematic review. J Clin Psychiatry 2006; 67:1836–1855.
10 Taylor D, Paton C, Kerwin R. The Maudsley Prescribing Guidelines, 9th edition. London: Informa Healthcare, 2007.
11 Rojo JE, Ros S, Aguera L, et al. Combined antidepressants: clinical experience. Acta Psychiatr Scand 2005; 112(Suppl 428):25–31.
12 Crossley NA, Bauer M. Acceleration and augmentation of antidepressants with lithium for depressive disorders: two meta-analyses of randomized, placebo-controlled trials. J Clin Psychiatry 2007; 68:935–940.
13 Papakostas GI, Shelton RC, Smith J, et al. Augmentation of antidepressants with atypical antipsychotic medications for treatment-resistant major depressive disorder: a meta-analysis. J Clin Psychiatry 2007; 68:826–831.
14 Thase ME, Friedman ES, Biggs MM, et al. Cognitive therapy versus medication in augmentation and switch strategies as second-step treatments: a STAR*D report. Am J Psychiatry 2007; 164:739–752.
15 Paykel ES, Scott J, Teasdale JD, et al. Prevention of relapse in residual depression by cognitive therapy. Arch Gen Psychiatry 1999; 56:829–835.
16 Pampallona S, Bollini P, Tibaldi G, et al. Combined pharmacotherapy and psychological treatment for depression: a systematic review. Arch Gen Psychiatry 2004; 61:714–719.
17 Thase ME, Greenhouse JB, Frank E, et al. Treatment of major depression with psychotherapy or psychotherapy-pharmacotherapy combinations. Arch Gen Psychiatry 1997; 54:1009–1015.

# Chapter 8

## Continuation and maintenance treatment

Ian M Anderson

As discussed in Chapter 4, the aim of the acute phase of treatment is remission. This chapter is concerned with treatment once this aim has been achieved.

### Goals of continuation/maintenance treatment

The goals of longer-term treatment are outlined in Chapter 4 and consist of continuing symptomatic and functional remission/recovery and consolidation and maintenance of wellbeing. A key point is preventing relapse/recurrence of depression and an important clinical issue is how long to advise continuing treatment beyond remission for individual patients. There are two aspects: continuing with treatment for as long as the benefits outweigh the risks/ adverse effects and minimizing risk factors for relapse/recurrence.

### Phases of treatment

An influential model of phases of treatment with antidepressants is that of Frank et al. (Figure 8.1) [1]. It proposes a continuum between depressive symptoms and major depression, with phases of treatment going through response to remission, which, if stable for 4–6 months, results in recovery. A return of depression is said to be a relapse before recovery and recurrence thereafter, and a distinction is made between continuation treatment to prevent relapse and maintenance treatment to prevent recurrence. The model has been helpful conceptually and in treatment trial design, but in practice it not possible to know when remission becomes recovery, so it is difficult to distinguish between relapse and recurrence. This is illustrated by ICD-10 requiring 2 months of absence of depressive symptoms to delineate different episodes, whereas DSM-IV requires only 2 months of not meeting major depression criteria. Neither of these agrees with the model in Figure 8.1, which requires 4–6 months of remission to define recovery.

E. Friedman and I.M. Anderson, *Managing Depression in Clinical Practice*
DOI 10.1007/978-1-84996-465-4_8, 

Model of treatment phases

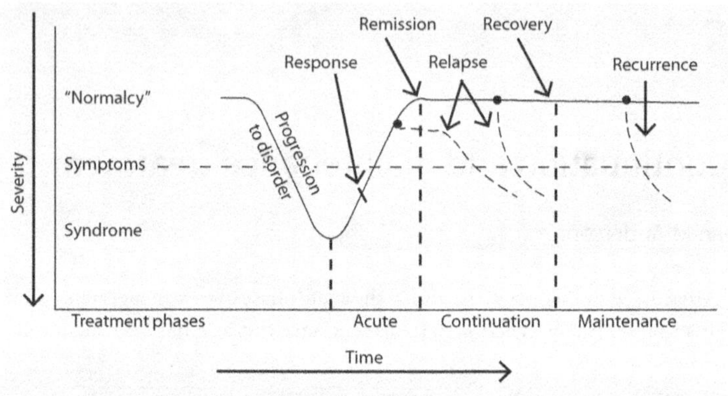


Figure 8.1 Model of treatment phases. Adapted with permission from [1].

An alternative is a continuum model based on the chance of a new episode of major depression over time after achievement of remission. Prospective studies show a high early rate of relapse, which gradually flattens out but never fully plateaus. The highest risk period is in the first 3 or 4 months with much lower risk beyond 1 year, but the risk varies depending on the individual's particular risk factors [2]. This influences the benefit that patients might receive from continuing treatment and therefore when to stop it.

## Medication

In patients with a relatively low risk of relapse (e.g., first episode), there is compelling evidence from placebo-controlled discontinuation studies that continuing antidepressants for a further 6–9 months after treatment prevents relapse (from approximately 50% to 20–25%) [3]. Beyond this time the risk of relapse is relatively low and the benefit from continuing antidepressants not apparent – this phase is often called the continuation phase after acute treatment and applicable to all patients whose depression remits with antidepressants.

In contrast, in highly recurrent depression (usually three episodes in the last 5 years) the benefit from antidepressants continues as long as the studies continue (the longest has been 5 years). The use of antidepressants after the continuation phase for prevention of further episodes of depression is often referred to as maintenance treatment. A meta-analysis of studies with follow-up as long as 3 years found that continuing antidepressants reduced the odds of relapse by 70%, irrespective of time from remission, even though the absolute risk of relapse was lower the greater the time since remission [4]. However, patients with recurrent depression who have done well on antidepressants still have a high risk of relapse even after 18 months' remission. A 2-year, randomized, placebo-controlled discontinuation study following 6 months' remission with open venlafaxine treatment found that, over 2 years, continuing venlafaxine reduced relapse to 29% from the 47% experienced on placebo. Most striking, however, were the results in patients who had remained well on venlafaxine over the first year and were re-randomized to continue venlafaxine or placebo. In the second year, only 7% of patients who remained on venlafaxine relapsed, compared with 37% on placebo [5].

The evidence for lithium being an effective maintenance treatment in unipolar depression is weaker than for antidepressants [6], but it is often used in specialist care in addition to antidepressants. If lithium has been used as an effective augmentation treatment it is usually best to continue this along with antidepressants to prevent relapse [7].

There has been debate about whether some antidepressants provide better protection against relapse/recurrence than others, in particular whether SSRIs lose efficacy. At present, the evidence is lacking as to whether this phenomenon exists or whether antidepressants differ in prophylactic efficacy. What is clear is that the treatment dose should be continued as the continuation and maintenance dose. There is no place for a lower "maintenance dose" of antidepressants because decreasing the treatment dose is associated with a higher risk of relapse [2].

Long-term treatment brings side effects more to the fore as patients who were willing to tolerate side effects to get better are usually less willing to put up with them long term when they are feeling well, particularly when they cause impairments in functioning and quality of life. It is therefore important to consider long-term side effects (e.g., sexual dysfunction and weight gain) when initially choosing treatment for patients who need maintenance treatment.

## Psychological treatments

Much less is known about continuation/maintenance treatment with psychological treatments. There is some evidence that initial successful treatment with CBT does provide protection against relapse after the treatment has finished [8]. This is in contrast to antidepressant treatment where continuing with treatment is required to prevent relapse. This makes CBT an important treatment option to consider in patients with recurrent depression because it has also been shown to be effective in relapse prevention when given to patients with a high recurrence risk after remission on antidepressants [9]. The presumed mechanism is the reduction of cognitive vulnerability to relapse through the techniques learned in therapy. However, recent studies suggest that relapse is delayed rather than prevented, and eventually patients do suffer another episode.

Continuation of CBT has been studied in one study, which found that 8 months' continuation treatment reduced relapse over that period in highly recurrent patients who had responded to CBT acutely. In the highest-risk groups (early onset and unstable remission in the acute phase) this benefit was maintained to 2 years [10]. In contrast, there is weaker evidence for relapse prevention with IPT and it is lacking with other forms of psychotherapy.

## Physical treatments

ECT (see Chapter 6) appears clinically useful as a continuation/maintenance treatment for a minority of patients who respond well to ECT but relapse occurs in spite of vigorous ongoing drug and psychological treatment [11]. In practice it is rare for patients to continue long term with ECT, but in individual cases it does not appear to cause cumulative cognitive or other adverse effects, or brain damage. The usual frequency of maintenance ECT is about monthly.

There is preliminary evidence that VNS (see Chapter 6) may reduce relapse in patients who have received benefits with acute treatment [12].

## Risk factors for relapse and recurrence

Figure 8.2 outlines factors that have been associated with higher risk of relapse or recurrence. The most important are probably the presence of residual symptoms, number of previous episodes, severity of index episode, and presence of treatment resistance (duration and degree of the most recent episode), but many of the factors clearly interact.

## Longer-term treatment in practice

Longer-term management of depression requires careful assessment of an individual's depressive disorder and risk of relapse. In addition, it is important to consider the consequences of relapse and the timing of withdrawal of antidepressant treatment because the risk of relapse is highest in the months after stopping or reducing the dose of antidepressants. It is difficult to predict with certainty and it is important to adopt a staged approach to the assessment of the need for continuing treatment, rather than set a fixed term. It often becomes clearer over time how high the risk is, with relapse or continuing symptoms making the need for treatment clearer.

It is best to approach the risk of recurrence as a continuum, taking into account the risk factors in Figure 8.2. The risks of relapse need to be discussed

| Risk factors associated with relapse/recurrence of depression |
|---|
| Shorter time since remission |
| Partial remission and residual symptoms |
| Number of previous episodes, especially two or more episodes in last 5 years |
| Severe index episode |
| Psychosis in index episode |
| Duration of symptoms, including dysthymia |
| Treatment resistance (duration and degree) |
| Persistence of social stress/poor social adjustment/life events |
| Comorbid physical illness |
| Comorbid anxiety |
| Female gender |
| Positive family history of depression |

Figure 8.2 Risk factors associated with relapse/recurrence of depression. Adapted from [2].

with patients as well as the risks and benefits of treatment, to help them make a considered decision about ongoing treatment. It is also important to help them consider the consequences of relapse and address any remedial risk factors for relapse (e.g., social stress, approaching life events, substance misuse), as well as lifestyle changes that might increase resilience to relapse (e.g., stable routines, exercise). Residual symptoms and cognitive factors for relapse (e.g., low self-esteem, negative self-evaluation, interpersonal sensitivity) are an indication to consider a specific psychotherapy (e.g., CBT) to consolidate remission.

Suggested starting points with regard to ongoing treatment [2]:

- After complete remission with antidepressant treatment in a patient with relatively low risk of recurrence (e.g., first episode depression in the absence of other risk factors), it is advisable to continue antidepressants for 6 months to prevent relapse.
- In patients with partial remission after antidepressant treatment or those with recurrent depression, undertaking CBT in addition to antidepressants is advisable to promote remission and reduce the risk of relapse.
- In patients with recurrent depression and unstable remission with CBT, a period of continuation CBT is advisable.
- In patients at significantly higher risk of relapse, who are in full or partial remission with antidepressant treatment, it is advisable to continue antidepressants and reassess after a minimum of 2 years' maintenance treatment. If a significant risk of relapse continues, then continuing antidepressants is advisable, if necessary indefinitely.

## References

1 Frank E, Prien RF, Jarrett RB, et al. Conceptualization and rationale for consensus definitions of terms in major depressive disorder. Remission, recovery, relapse, and recurrence. Arch Gen Psychiatry 1991, 48:851–855.
2 Anderson I, Ferrier I, Baldwin R, et al. Evidence-based guidelines for treating depressive disorders with antidepressants: a revision of the 2000 British Association for Psychopharmacology guidelines. J Psychopharmacol 2008; 22:343–396.
3 Reimherr FW, Amsterdam JD, Quitkin FM. Optimal length of continuation therapy in depression: a prospective assessment during long term fluoxetine treatment. Am J Psychiatry 1998; 155:1247–1253.
4 Geddes JR, Carney SM, Davies C, et al. Relapse prevention with antidepressant drug treatment in depressive disorders: a systematic review. Lancet 2003; 361:653–661.
5 Keller MB, Trivedi MH, Thase ME, et al. The prevention of recurrent episodes of depression with venlafaxine for two years (PREVENT) study: outcomes from the 2-year and combined maintenance phases. J Clin Psychiatry 2007; 68:1246–1256.
6 Burgess S, Geddes J, Hawton K, et al. Lithium for maintenance treatment of mood disorders. Cochrane Database Syst Rev 2001; CD003013.
7 Bauer M, Bschor T, Kunz D, et al. Double-blind, placebo-controlled trial of the use of lithium to augment antidepressant medication in continuation treatment of unipolar major depression. Am J Psychiatry 2000; 157:1429–1435.
8 Hensley PL, Nadiga D, Uhlenhuth EH. Long-term effectiveness of cognitive therapy in major depressive disorder. Depress Anxiety 2004; 20:1–7.
9 Paykel ES. Cognitive therapy in relapse prevention in depression. Int J Neuropsychopharmacol 2007; 10:131–136.
10 Jarrett RB, Kraft D, Doyle J, et al. Preventing recurrent depression using cognitive therapy with and without a continuation phase: a randomized clinical trial. Arch Gen Psychiatry 2001; 58:381–388.
11 Gagne GG, Jr., Furman MJ, Carpenter LL, et al. Efficacy of continuation ECT and antidepressant drugs compared to long-term antidepressants alone in depressed patients. Am J Psychiatry 2000; 157:1960–1965.
12 Sackeim HA, Brannan SK, John RA, et al. Durability of antidepressant response to vagus nerve stimulation (VNSTM). Int J Neuropsychopharmacol 2007; 10:817–826.

# Index

Made in United States
Cleveland, OH
27 September 2026

44872774R00066